# Nature of Beauty:
## The Surprising Origins of Natural Cosmetic Ingredients

Valerie J. Reed

ISBN: 10:1548805327
ISBN-13:978 -1548805326

Contact: service@valanaminerals.com
Visit: valanaminerals.com and ur.valanaminerals.com

# ACKNOWLEDGMENTS

For my mentor and friend, Dee, who believed in me even when I was unsure of myself, my husband Dean, brother Nathan and parents Charles and Andrea, whose help and support foster my creativity.

# Contents

# Section 1

The Minerals, Metals & Gems

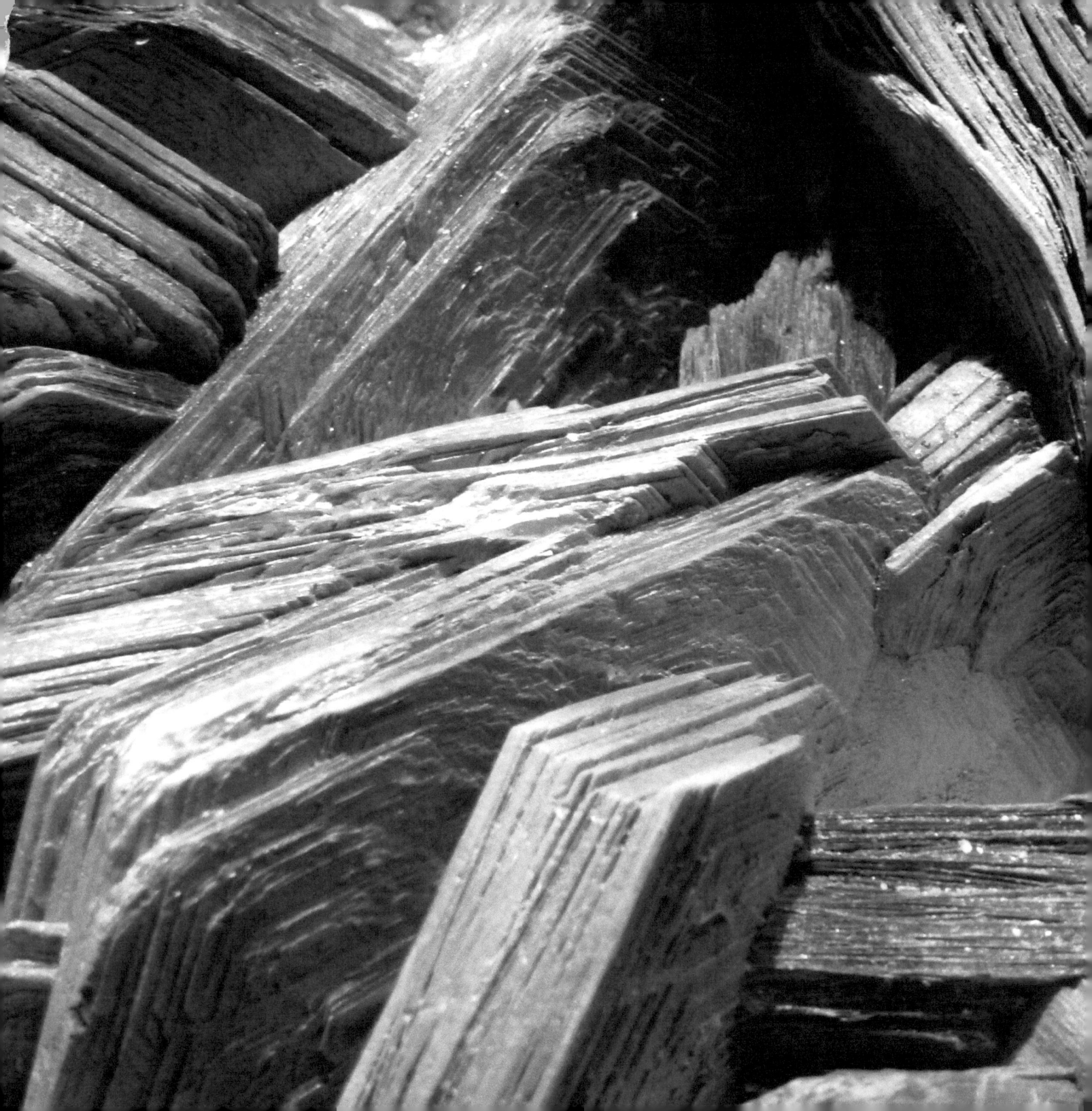

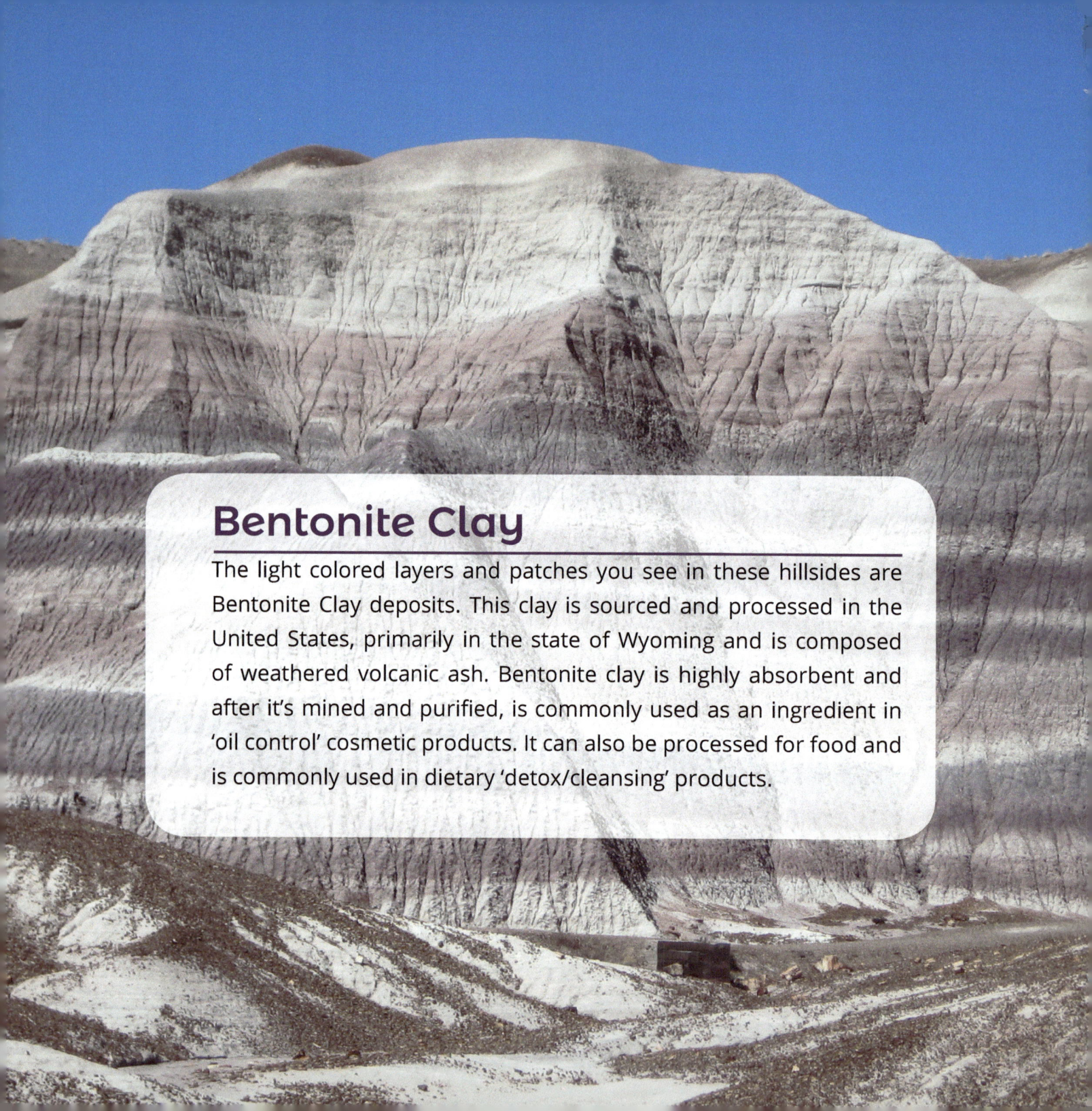

# Bentonite Clay

The light colored layers and patches you see in these hillsides are Bentonite Clay deposits. This clay is sourced and processed in the United States, primarily in the state of Wyoming and is composed of weathered volcanic ash. Bentonite clay is highly absorbent and after it's mined and purified, is commonly used as an ingredient in 'oil control' cosmetic products. It can also be processed for food and is commonly used in dietary 'detox/cleansing' products.

# Gold

This metal is soft compared to other metals. Gold tends to be yellow in color and is mined from the earth's crust. Gold may add to the feeling of luxury to cosmetic products. Glitter flecks, powdered and dispersed in liquid are just a couple of the ways you might notice gold in your cosmetics. Gold powder and film is also used in food; yes, people eat gold.

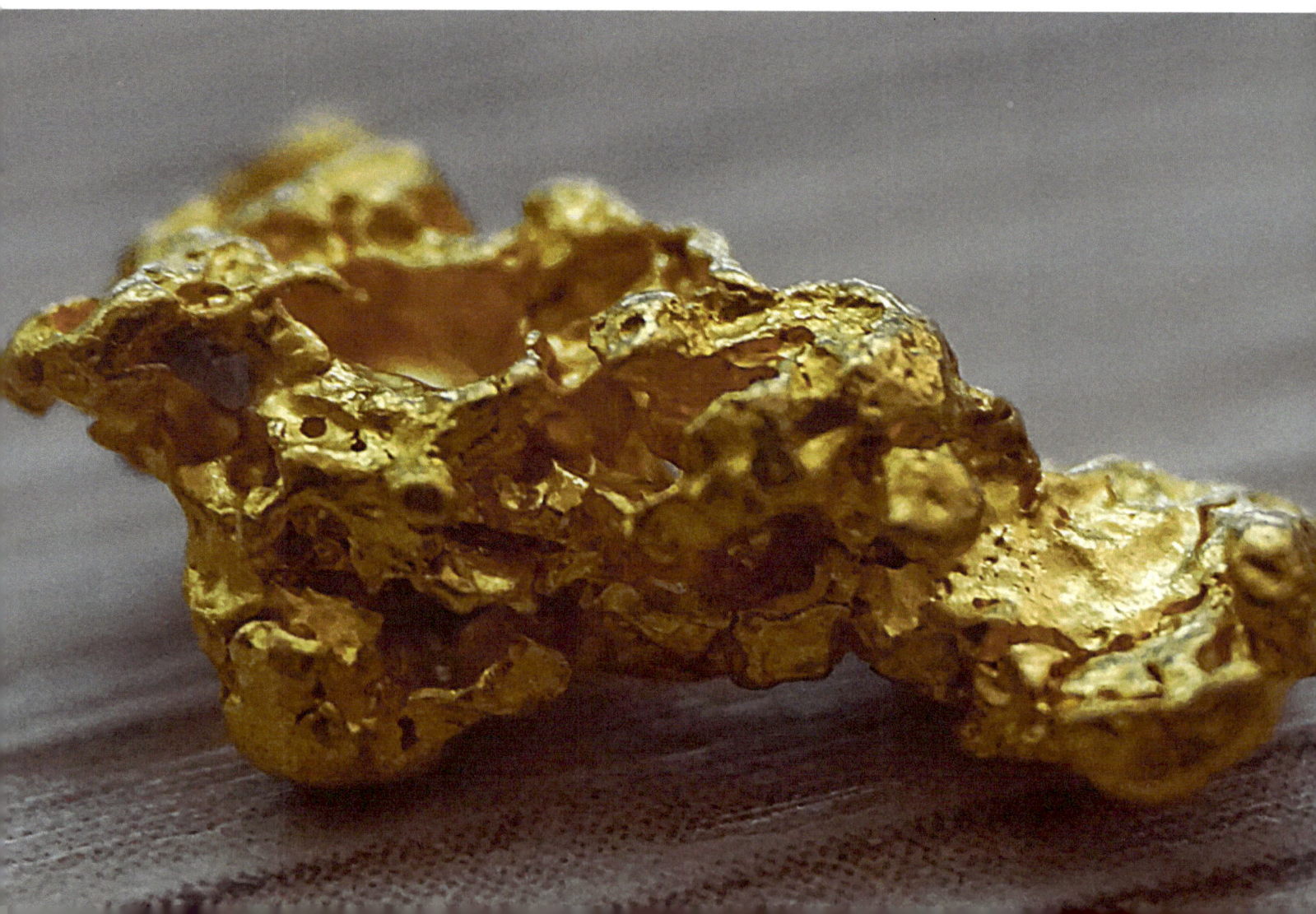

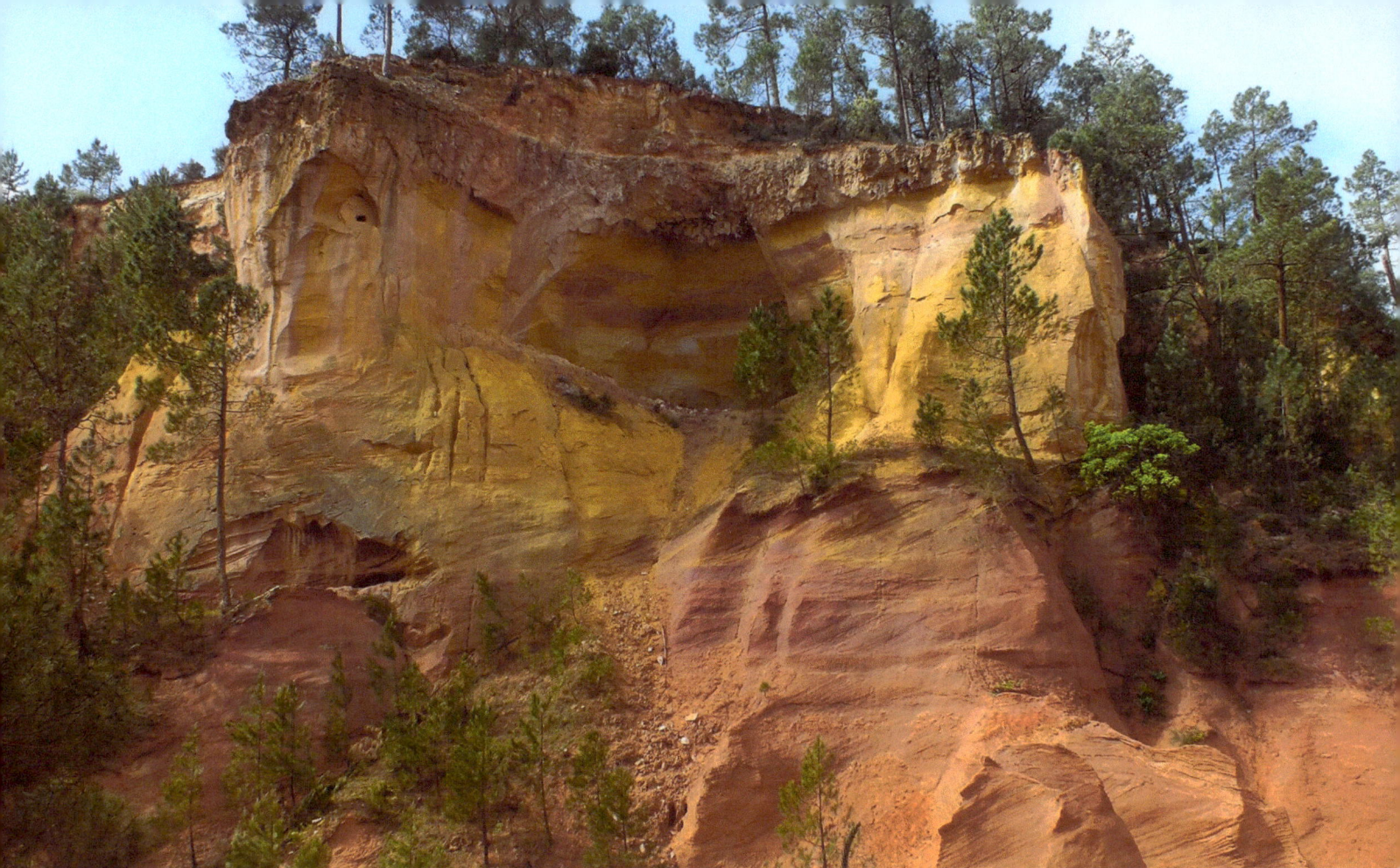

# Iron Oxides

Oxygen, water and heat combined with iron gives us, iron oxides. Iron oxides can be processed into many different shades. The resulting color varies depending on the temperature at which its processed. In this image the red striations in the hillside are red iron oxides while the deep golden layers are a variation of iron oxide called ochre. Iron Oxides are commonly used in color cosmetics in the form of matte powder. They may also be processed for use as food coloring.

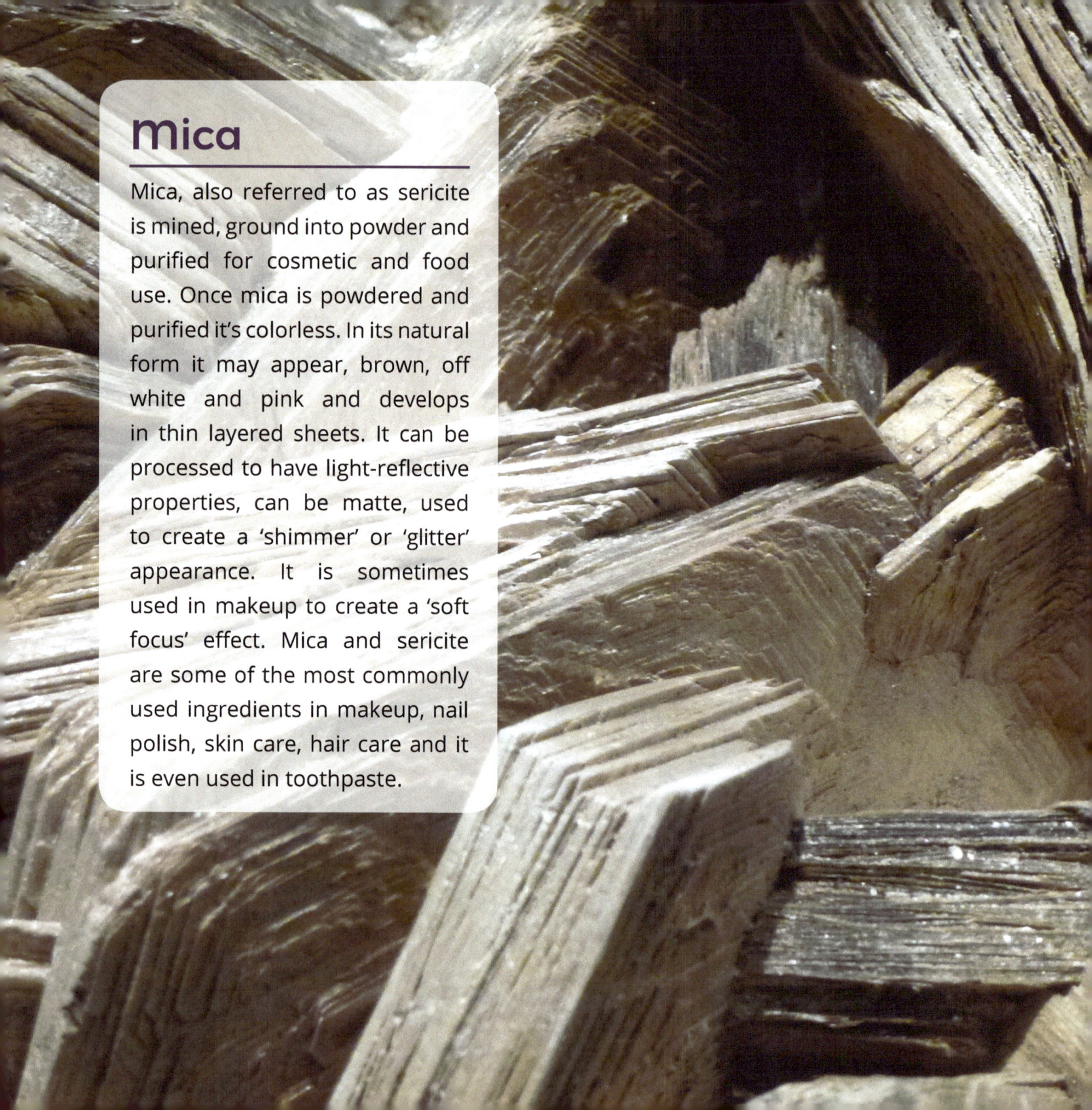

# mica

Mica, also referred to as sericite is mined, ground into powder and purified for cosmetic and food use. Once mica is powdered and purified it's colorless. In its natural form it may appear, brown, off white and pink and develops in thin layered sheets. It can be processed to have light-reflective properties, can be matte, used to create a 'shimmer' or 'glitter' appearance. It is sometimes used in makeup to create a 'soft focus' effect. Mica and sericite are some of the most commonly used ingredients in makeup, nail polish, skin care, hair care and it is even used in toothpaste.

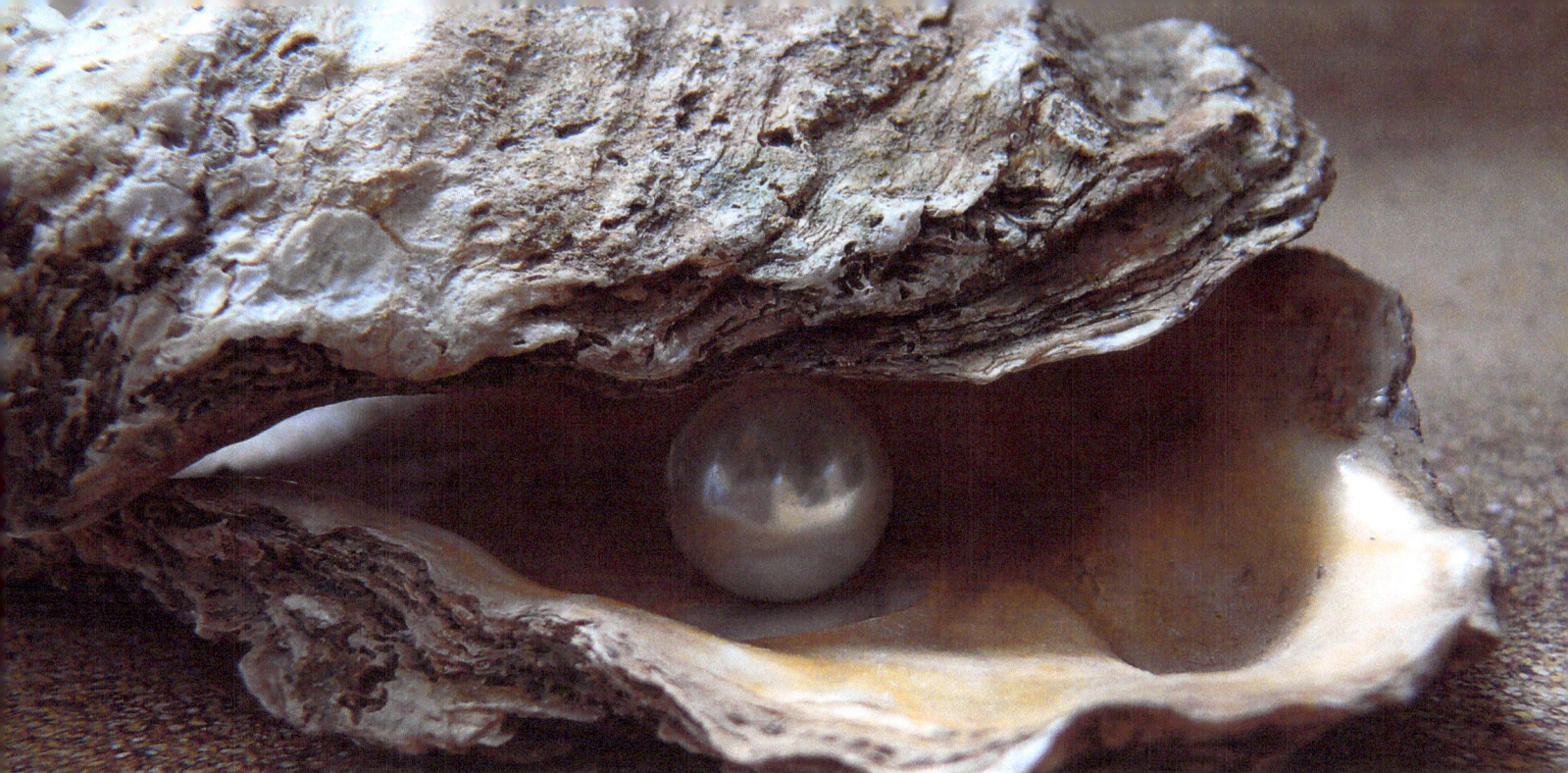

# Pearls

The process that an oyster undergoes to produce a pearl can occur naturally or may be farmed. The process involves an irritant, like a grain of sand or a parasite entering or being implanted inside the oyster, mussel or clam shell. In response to the irritant, the oyster, mussel or clam produces a fluid called nacre (made of calcium) as a defense or protection from the irritant (grain of sand or parasite). The nacre forms a coating around the irritant. After a few years the layers of nacre build up, forming a pearl. For cosmetic use pearls are farmed, harvested and ground into a fine powder. Pearl powder tends to be matte (no shine at all) off white color and contains approximately 15 different amino acids and 10 different minerals. It's often used in skin care creams and anti-aging cosmetics.

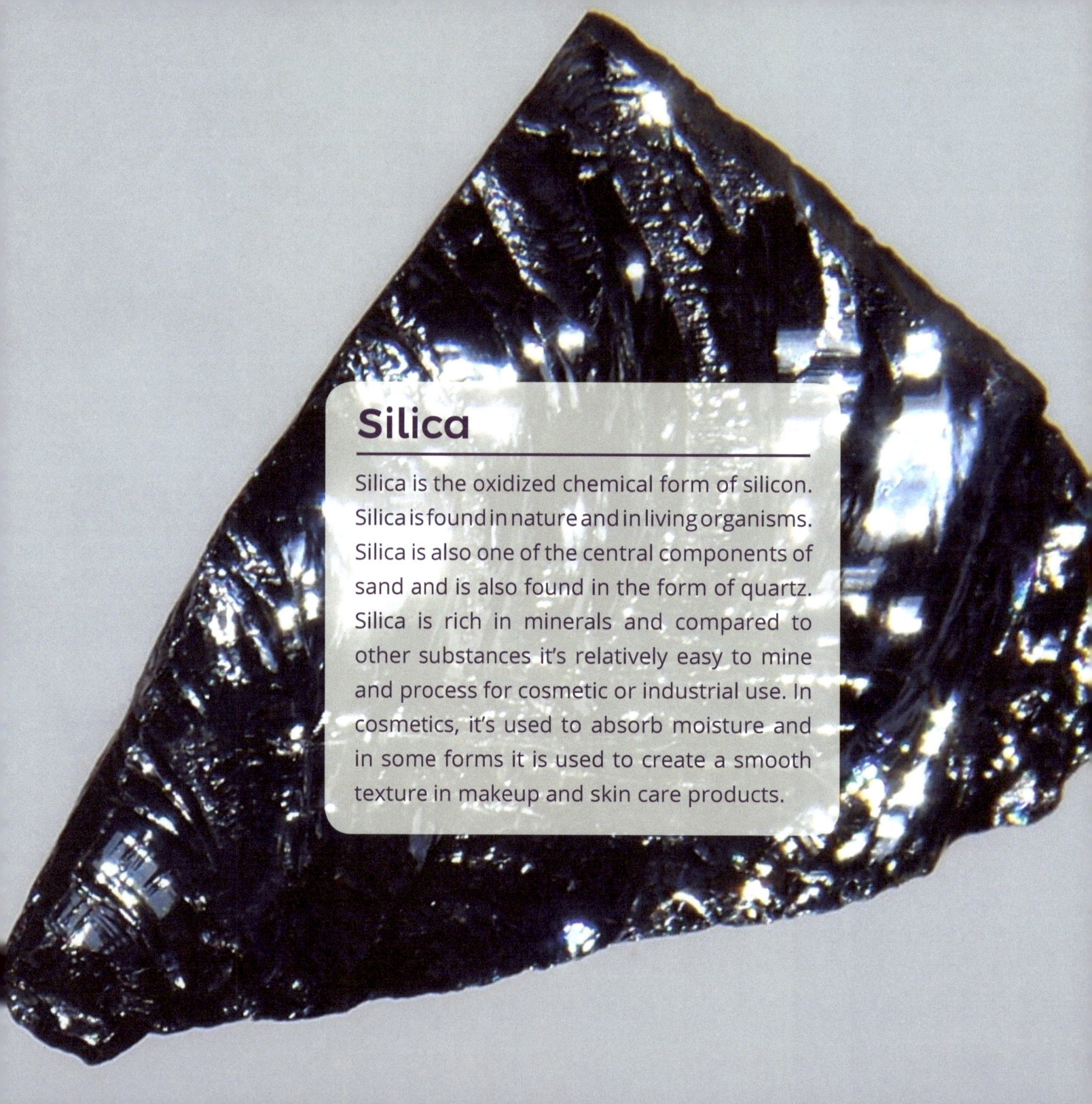

# Silica

Silica is the oxidized chemical form of silicon. Silica is found in nature and in living organisms. Silica is also one of the central components of sand and is also found in the form of quartz. Silica is rich in minerals and compared to other substances it's relatively easy to mine and process for cosmetic or industrial use. In cosmetics, it's used to absorb moisture and in some forms it is used to create a smooth texture in makeup and skin care products.

# Silver

A soft, white or gray metal that is mined for use in cosmetics and in medicinal products. In medicinal products, it's used as a germicide, while in cosmetics it is used as a coloring, typically in nail polish, mouthwash or as a luxury additive in skin care creams and ointments. It can be quite irritating to the skin and result in allergic reactions.

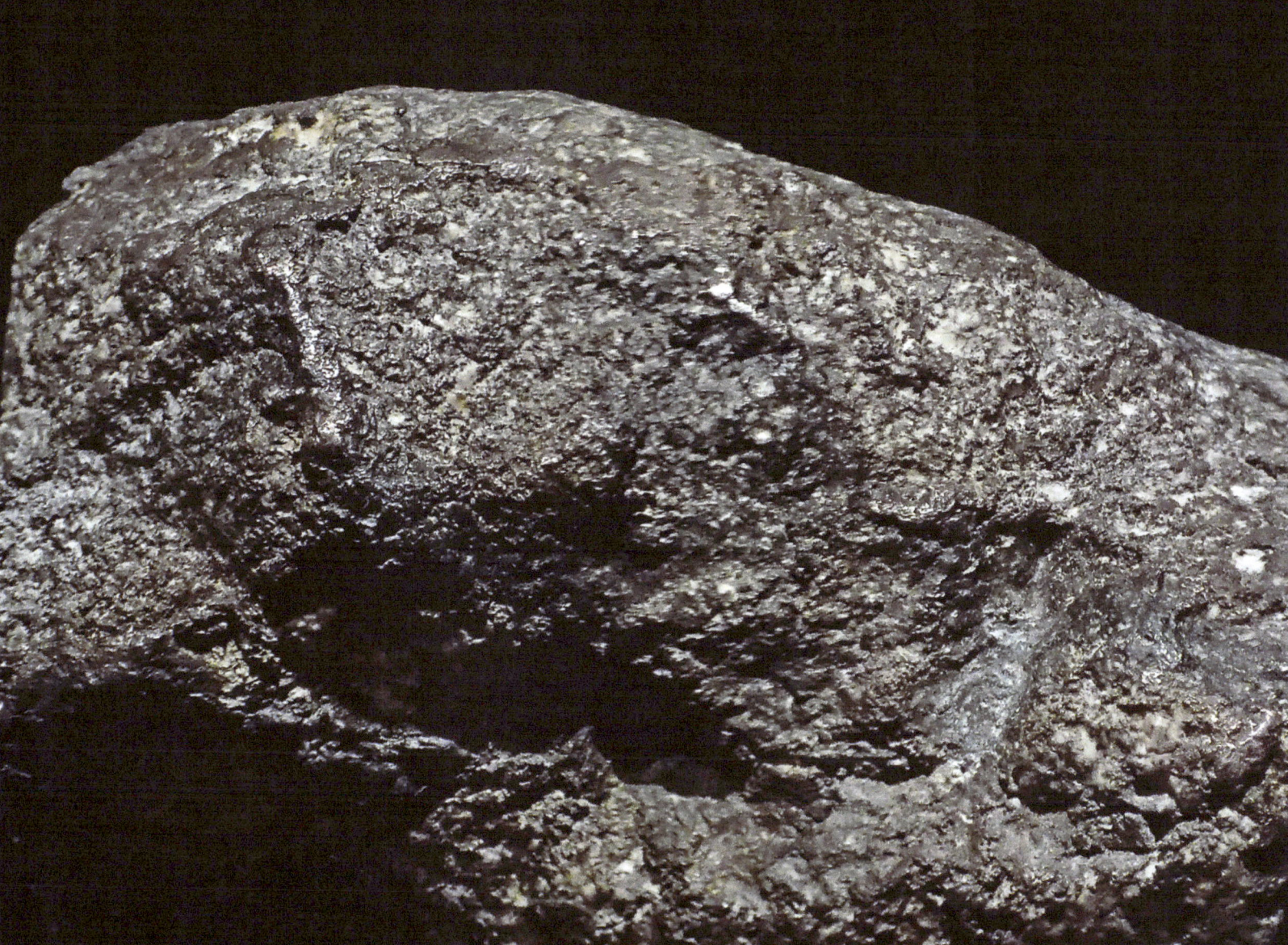

# Section 2

The Animals, Insects & a Mollusk

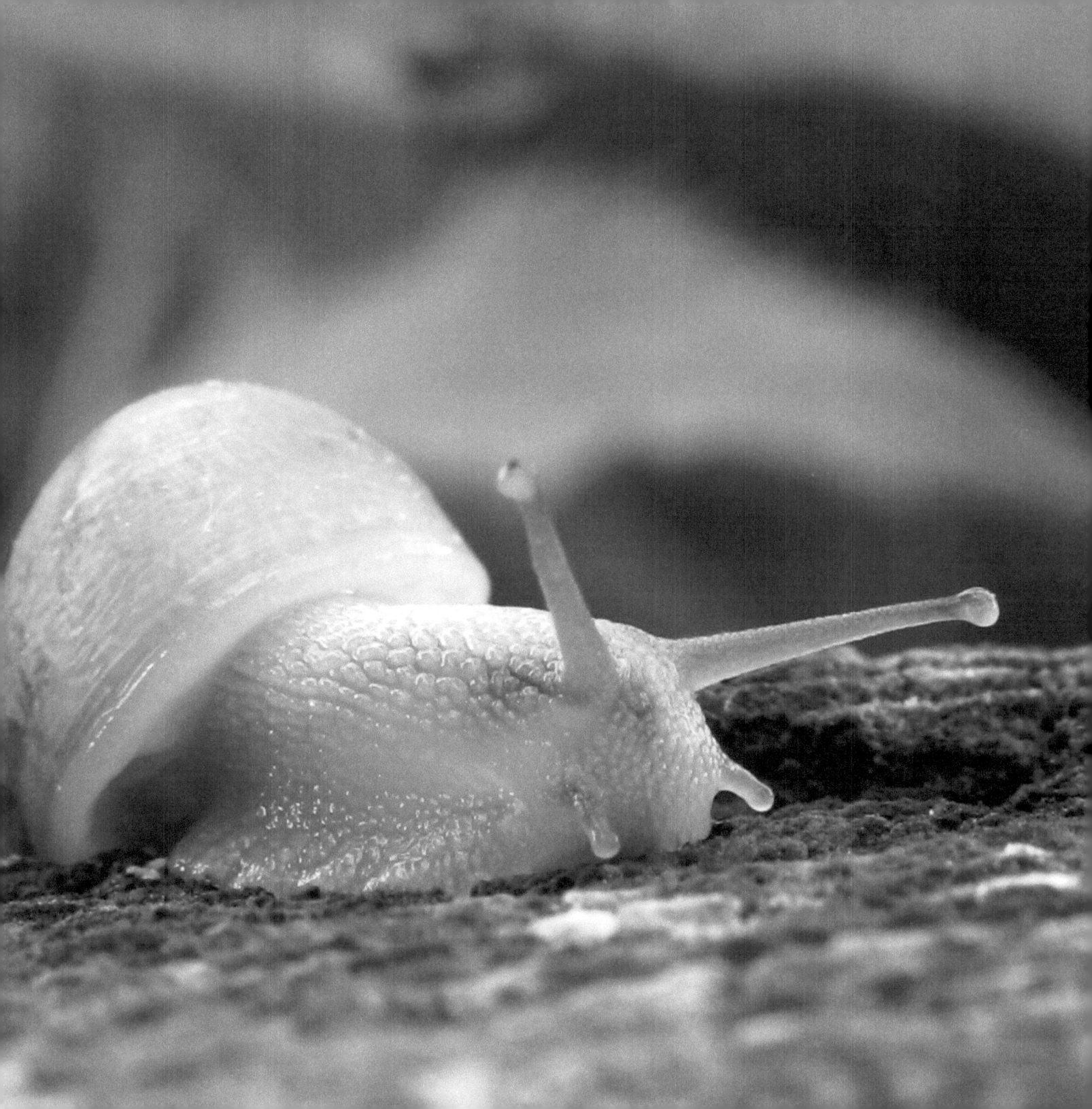

# Bees

The fact that bees produce honey and beeswax is not the the surprising part here. How the bees produce honey and beeswax, however, is fascinating. The lifespan of a worker bee is about a month. During their short lives they work constantly collecting nectar or pollen (each worker bee carries only one load at a time, either pollen or nectar but not both) to return to the hive. Bees that collect nectar store it in their storage stomach and some is used for their fuel. When the nectar is in the storage stomach it mixes with an enzyme and begins it's transformation into honey. When the nectar carrying bees return to the hive, they regurgitate the nectar/honey into the mouths of the receiver bees where the nectar/honey mixes with more enzymes. The receiver bees then deposit the nectar/honey into comb cavities of the hive. Over time, the liquid goes through an evaporation process to completely transform into honey. Bees consume honey and mix honey and pollen, which is used to feed new generations of bees.

Worker bees consume honey. The digestive process of the bees consuming honey results in the bees producing wax scales on their bodies. Worker bees have glands in their bodies that extrude the wax scales. Other bees remove the wax scales from their hive-mates, chew the wax then use it to build the hexagon shaped combs. This also explains why unrefined beeswax smells and tastes like honey. The combs are used to store honey and the next generation of bees. Bees consume about seven pounds of honey to make one pound of beeswax.

Both honey and beeswax have been used in cosmetics for centuries and are commonly used in cosmetic products today. Honey is a humectant so it's often used in moisturizing cosmetic products such as, moisturizers, hair conditioners, facial masks and lip conditioners. Beeswax is used as a thickener and stabilizer in lipsticks, lip glosses, lip balms, moisturizing creams, hair conditioners and makeup products.

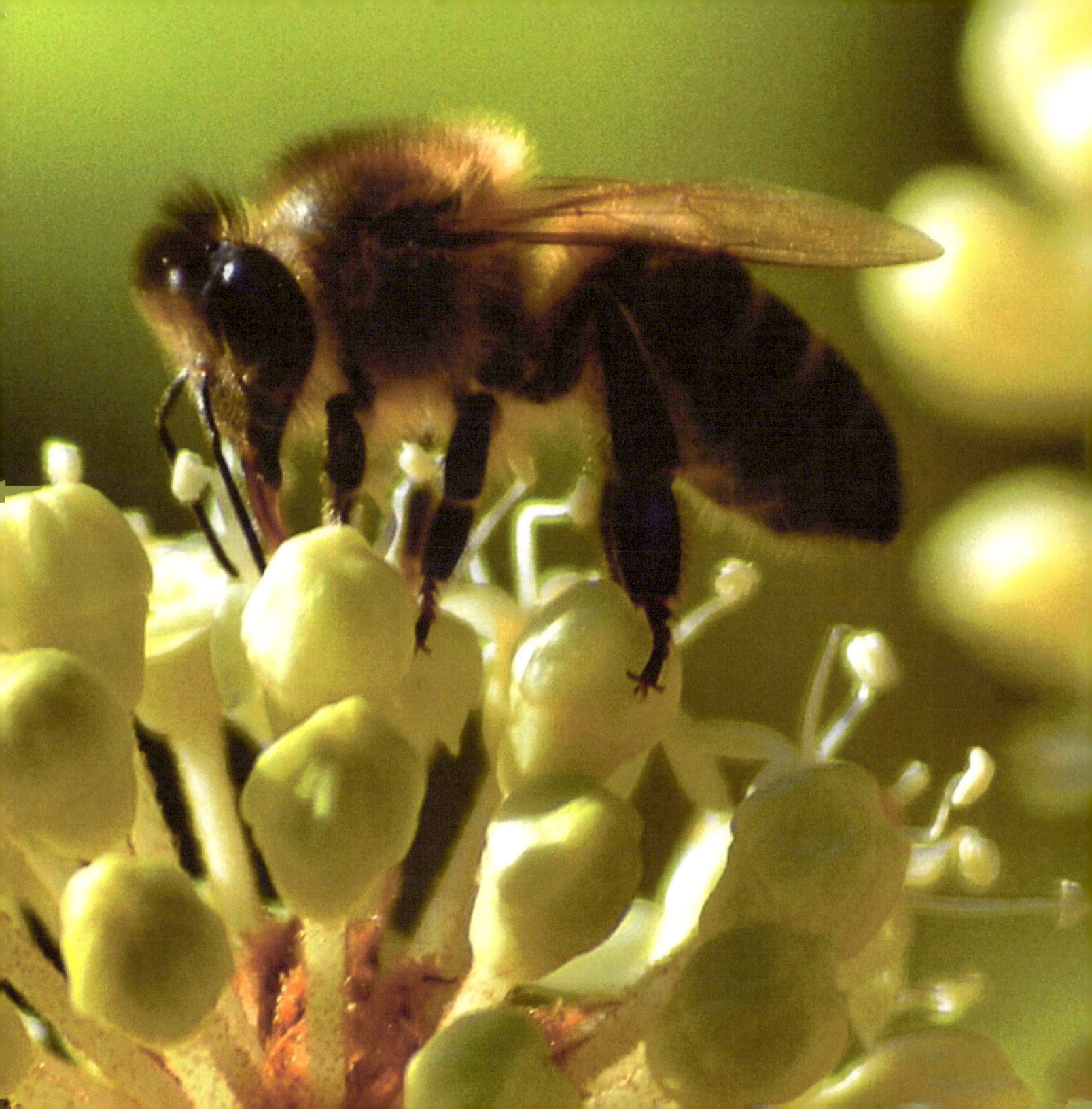

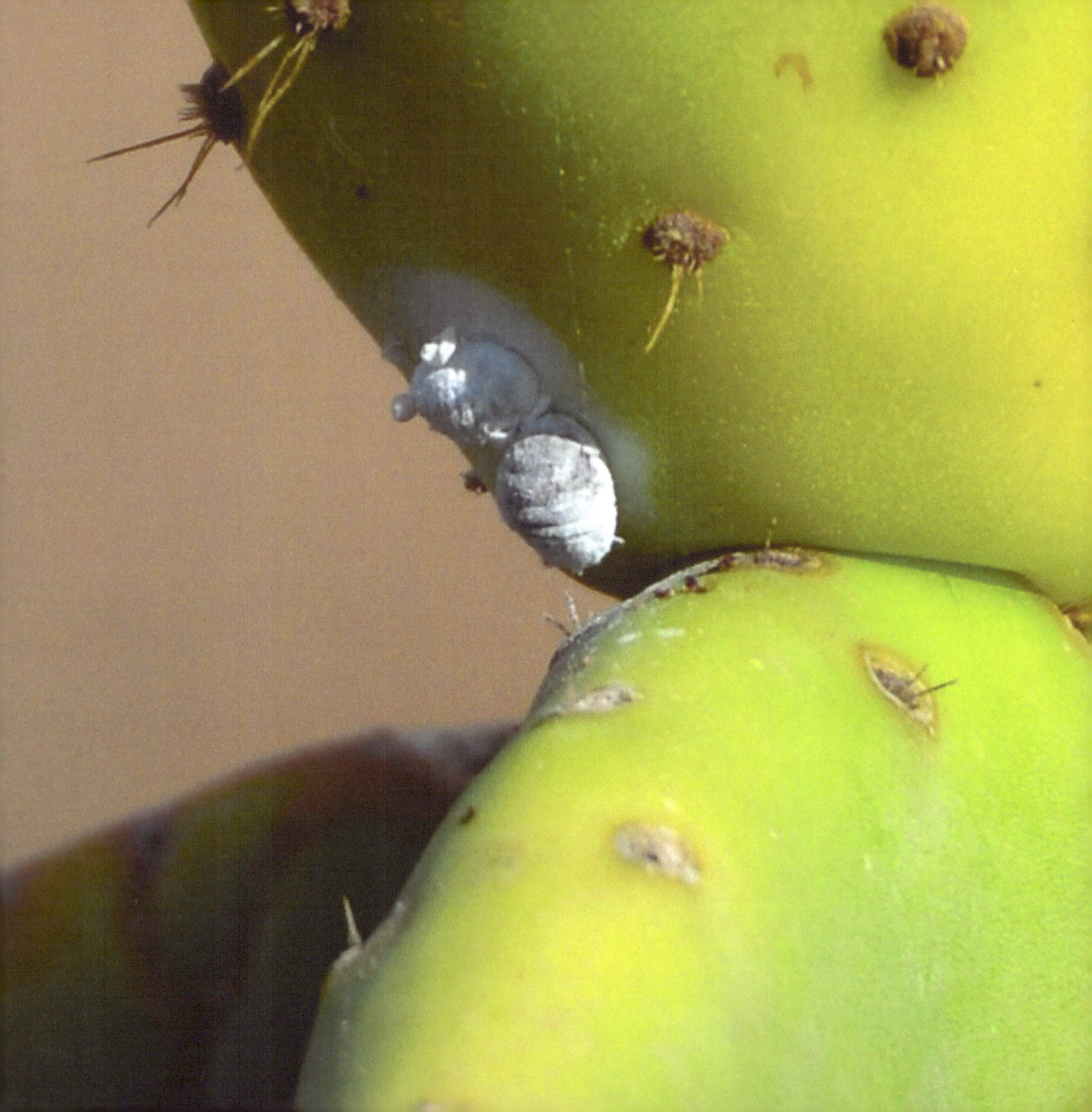

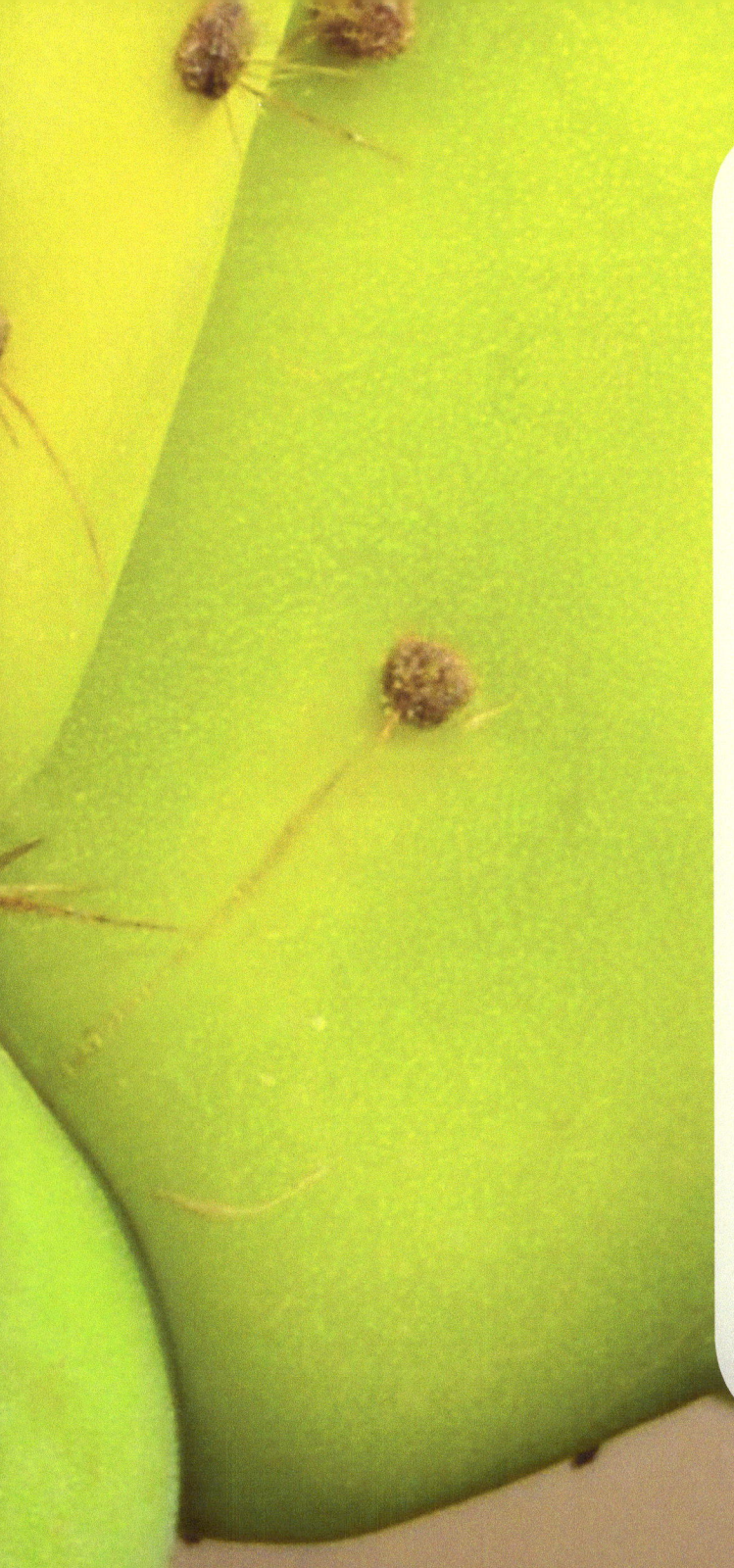

# Cochineal Beetles

Carmine is a red pigment/dye that is produced from the shell or exoskeleton and eggs of the female Cochineal Beetle. The beetle is commonly found in Arizona, Mexico and some areas of Central and South America. The Cochineal beetle lives on and in cactus. The beetles are harvested and dried. In some form or another carmine has been used as dye for hundreds of years. The modern process involves mixing cultivated or farmed, dried exoskeleton and eggs with aluminum, calcium salt and other ingredients to produce the dye, which ends up being an extract of the beetle. Cosmetics and food manufacturers in the United States are permitted to use Cochineal Beetle extract. Carmine is used to produce dye in cosmetics such as eyeshadow and lipstick and many other make-up products and nail polishes. It's also used as a food dye. Photo: The white, fuzzy looking clusters at the base of the prickly pear fruit on the cactus are Cochineal beetles.

# Racoon, Pony, Squirrel, Siberian Weasel (sable) and Badger

The majority of cosmetic brushes available today are made with various types of animal hair or fur. Synthetic cosmetic brushes are more easily available and the quality is better now than previously. Nevertheless, animal hair brushes dominate the cosmetic market. Animals are farmed for their hair or fur. The butchering process may render the carcass for other uses, while the pelt and/or tail is used to gather hair or fur. Cosmetic brushes labeled only "natural bristles" typically have a mix of different types of animal hair or are from animals that people generally aren't in favor of farming or butchering.

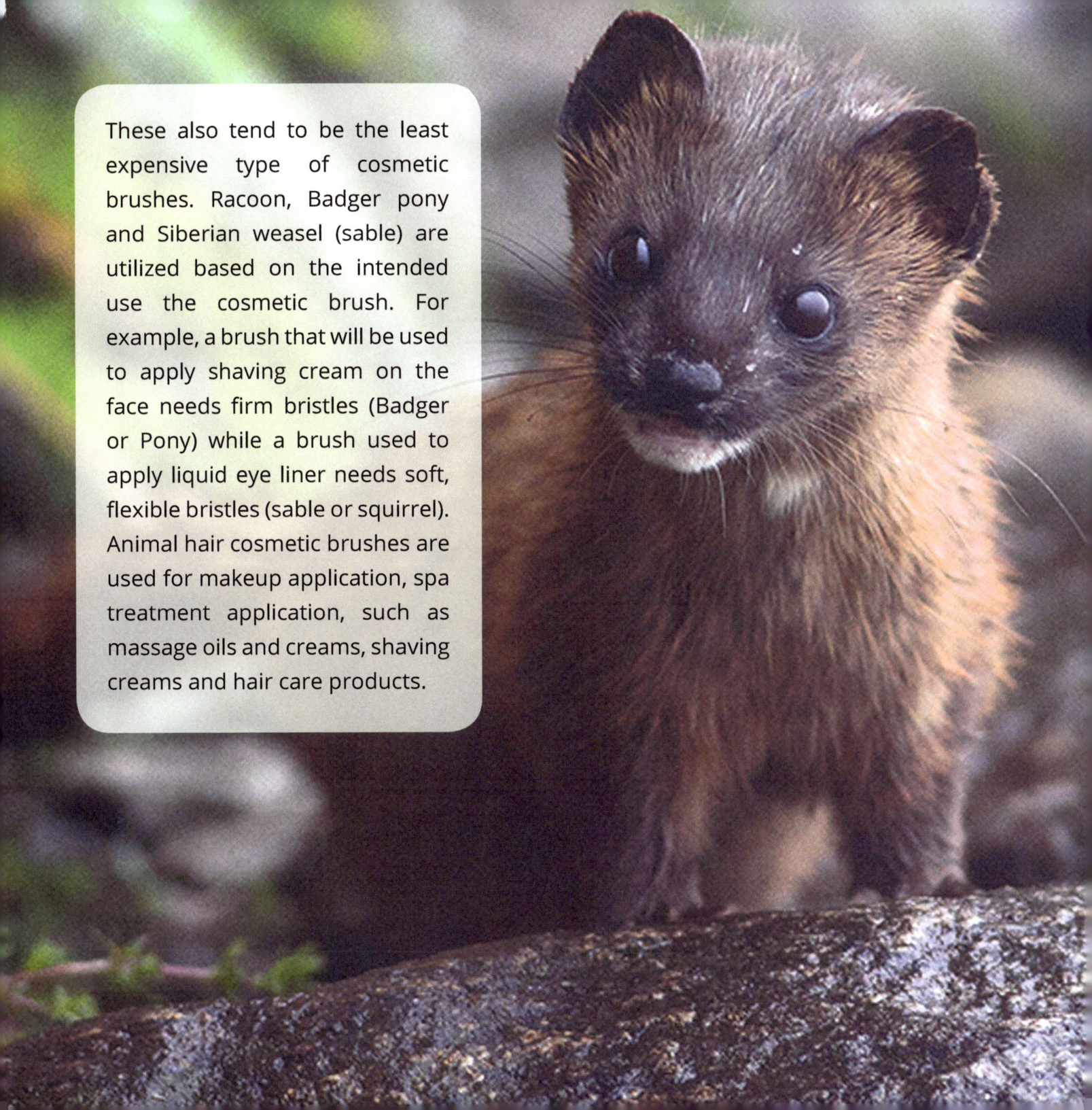

These also tend to be the least expensive type of cosmetic brushes. Racoon, Badger pony and Siberian weasel (sable) are utilized based on the intended use the cosmetic brush. For example, a brush that will be used to apply shaving cream on the face needs firm bristles (Badger or Pony) while a brush used to apply liquid eye liner needs soft, flexible bristles (sable or squirrel). Animal hair cosmetic brushes are used for makeup application, spa treatment application, such as massage oils and creams, shaving creams and hair care products.

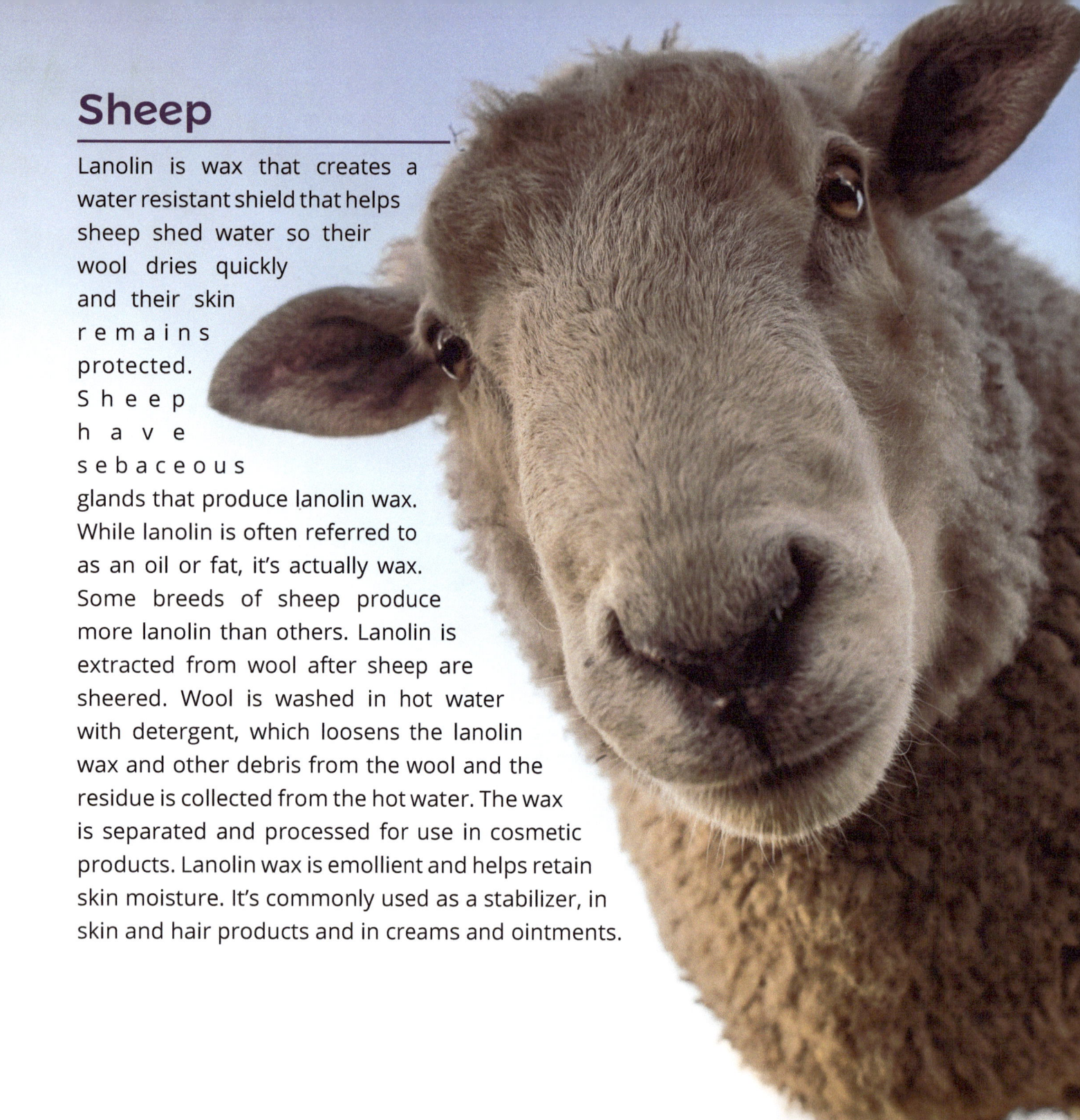

# Sheep

Lanolin is wax that creates a water resistant shield that helps sheep shed water so their wool dries quickly and their skin remains protected. Sheep have sebaceous glands that produce lanolin wax. While lanolin is often referred to as an oil or fat, it's actually wax. Some breeds of sheep produce more lanolin than others. Lanolin is extracted from wool after sheep are sheered. Wool is washed in hot water with detergent, which loosens the lanolin wax and other debris from the wool and the residue is collected from the hot water. The wax is separated and processed for use in cosmetic products. Lanolin wax is emollient and helps retain skin moisture. It's commonly used as a stabilizer, in skin and hair products and in creams and ointments.

# Snails

Snail slime or snail filtrate has been used in cosmetic products for generations. Snails secrete fluid called mucin, which is primarily comprised of water but a small proportion of mucin contains hyaluronic acid and glycoproteins and other components considered beneficial for human skin. Today common garden snails are cultivated or farmed under controlled conditions and mucin is harvested and processed into snail filtrate for use in cosmetics. Snail filtrate is most commonly used in anti-aging and moisturizing cosmetic products.

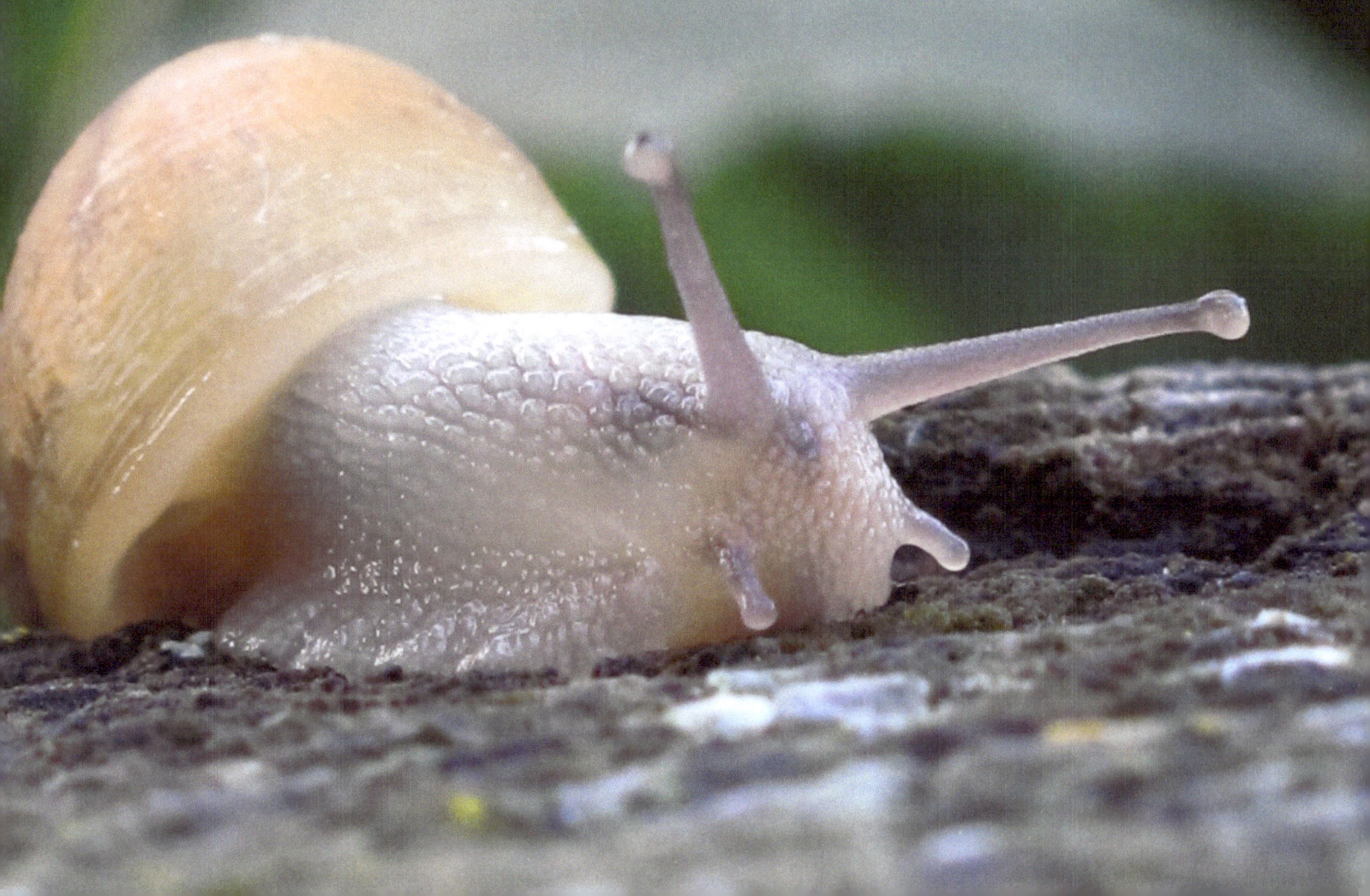

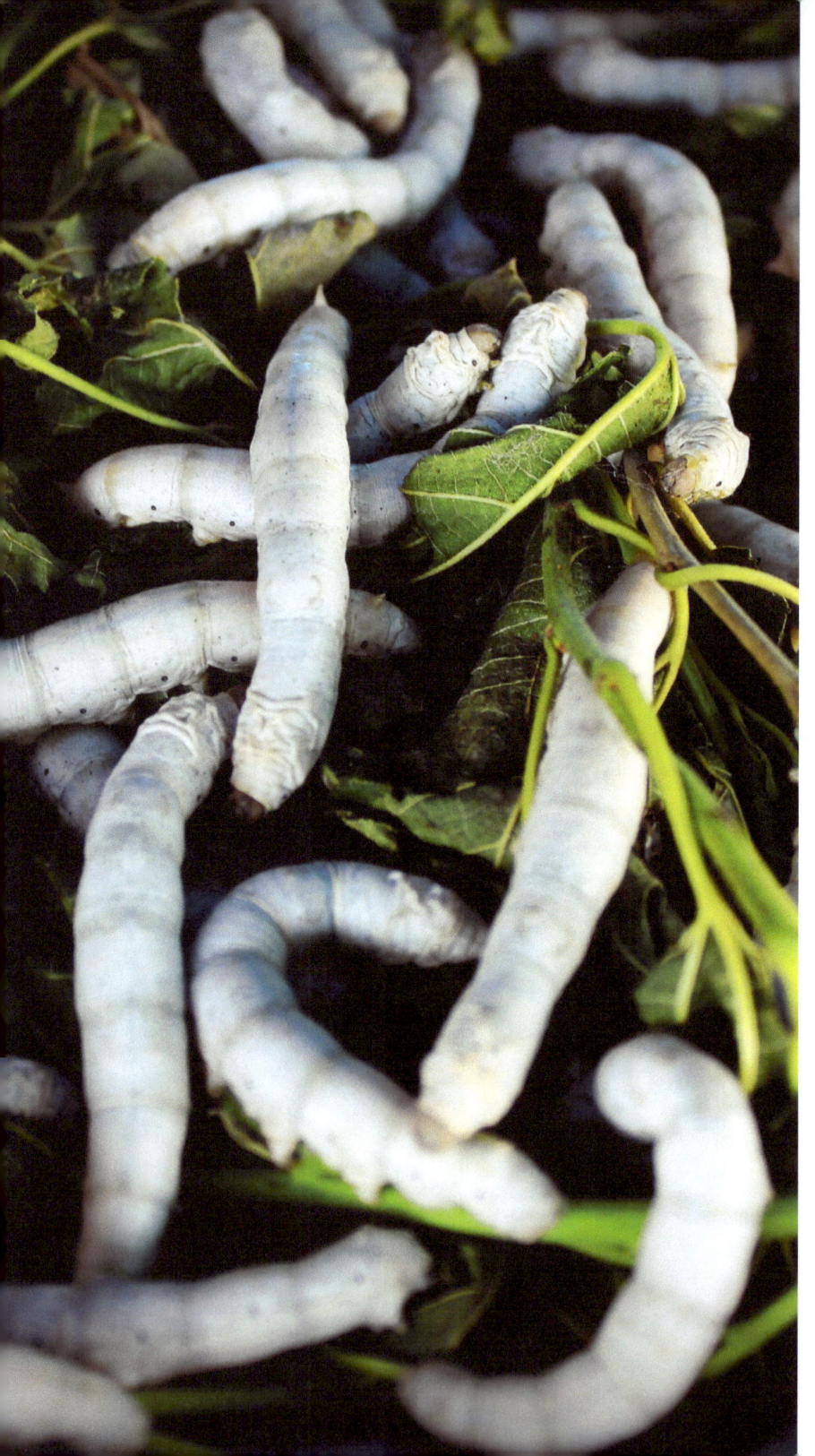

# Silk

Certain types of caterpillars or larvae produce protein fiber, called silk, during the process of creating their cocoon to undergo metamorphosis from larvae to moth. There are also some types of crickets, wasps, beetles and other insects that produce protein fiber, but these aren't used in silk production. The moth caterpillar is the type most commonly harvested for silk production and manufacturing. Silk production has a long history throughout China, South Asia, Middle East, Africa, South America and later in North America. Silk can be farmed-cultivated or wild harvested. When the moth caterpillar or larvae prepares to create a cocoon, it excretes a long thread of protein fiber, in which the moth caterpillar surrounds itself, thus constructing its cocoon.

In farmed or cultivated settings the cocoon is harvested and processed so that the larvae caterpillar dies inside the cocoon and the long, continuous protein filament thread can be retrieved intact and can be as long as 1,000 feet in length. Wild harvested cocoons tend to have irregular or broken protein filament threads because they are retrieved after the larvae caterpillar has become a moth and has broken through the cocoon. Intact silk filament thread is more costly than broken, or wild harvested threads. For cosmetic use, silk is, dried and milled into a fine powder. Silk powder is used in cosmetics to retain skin moisture, absorb oil and to create a soft focus effect in makeup finishing products.

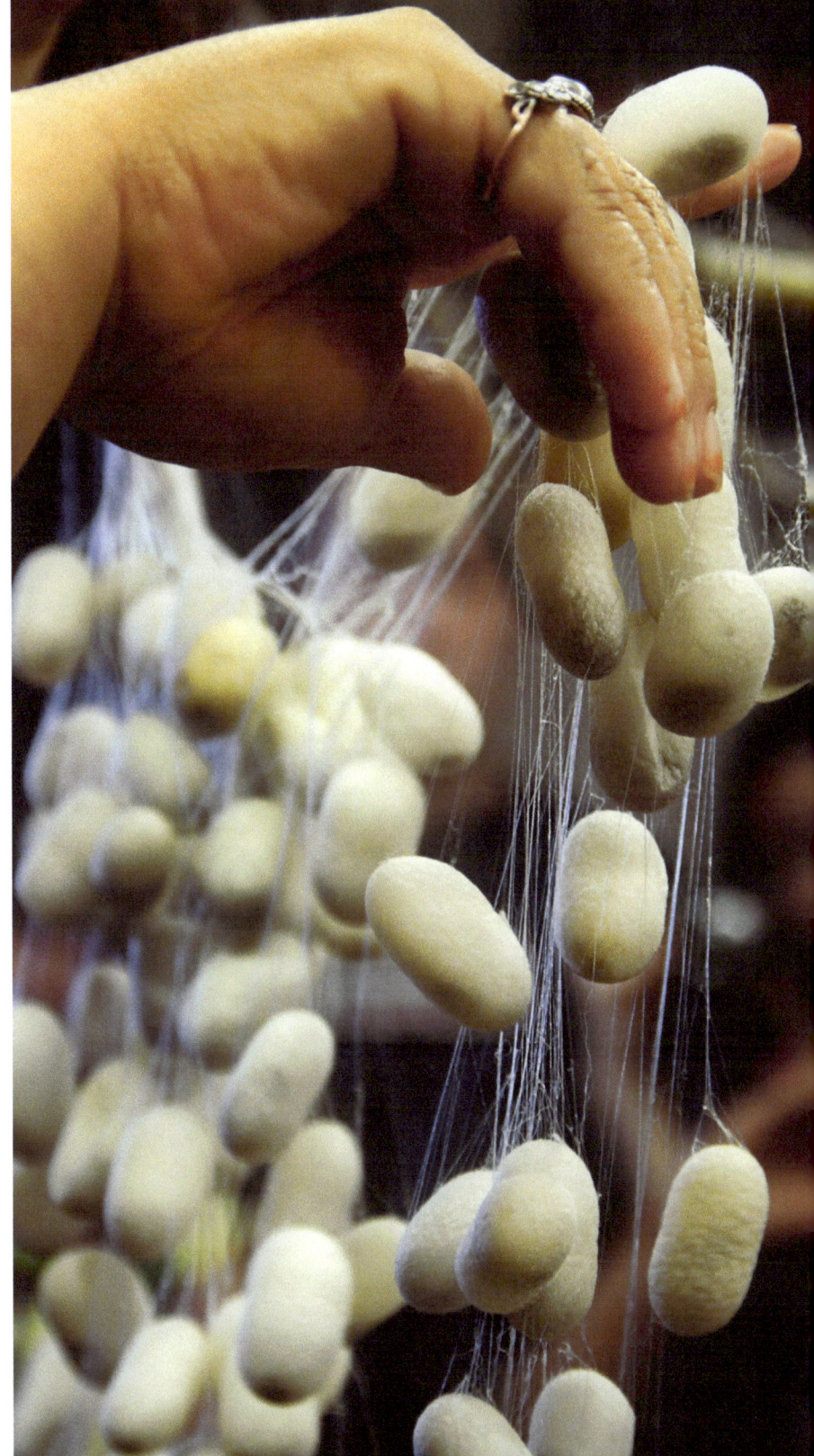

# Section 3

## The Plants

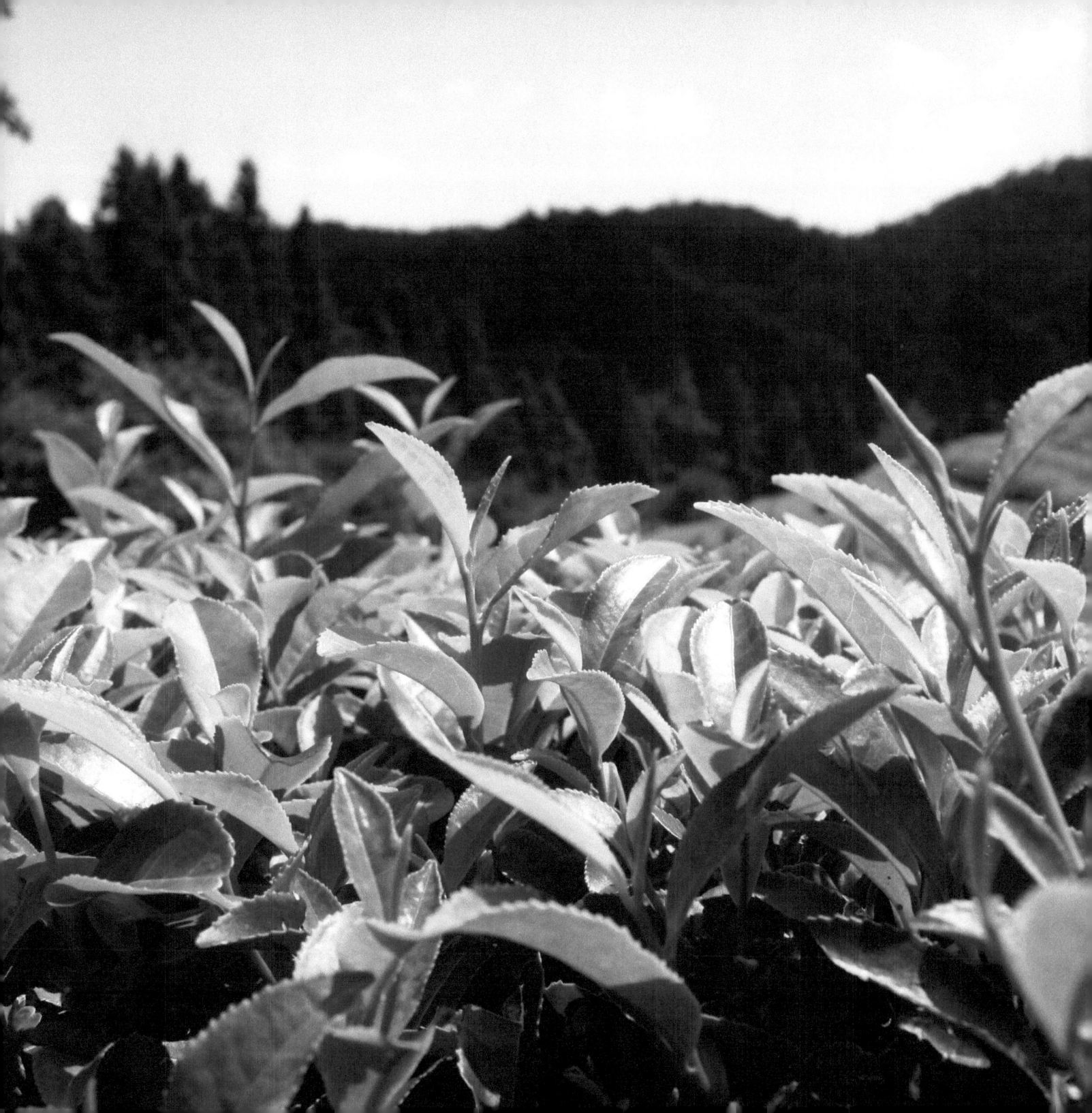

# Bananas

Bananas that aren't pretty enough to be sold to grocery stores can be processed into gluten free flour, starch or fragrance. Banana flour and starch is used as a thickener and stabilizer in cosmetic products. Fragrance made from "waste" bananas can be used in food and is also used in lip color and lip balm products.

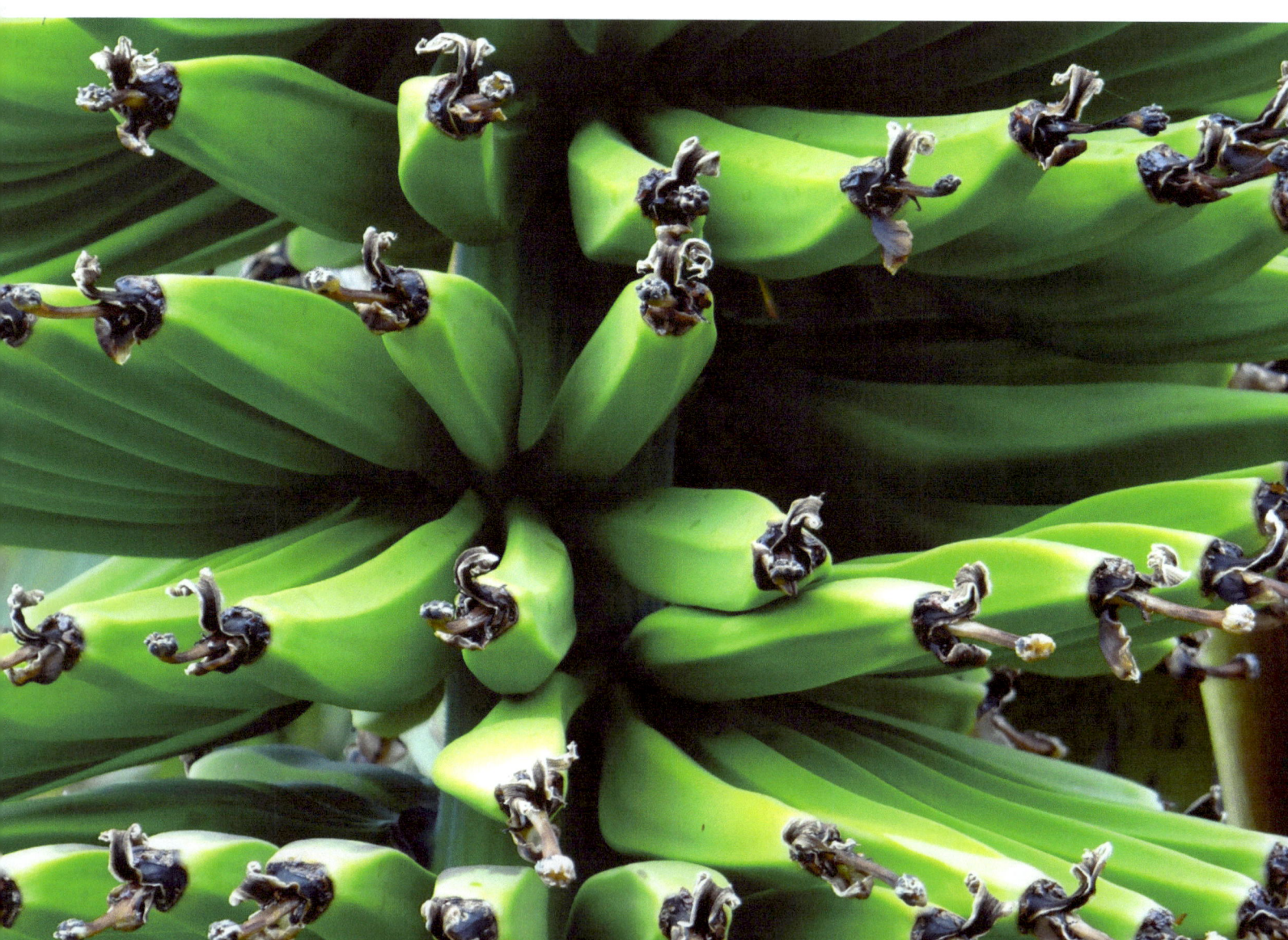

# Candellila

This is a light-yellow plant-based wax. The plant grows in clusters and can grow to about three feet tall. The wax forms on the stalks and looks like a coating of yellowish scales. Horses and donkeys like to nibble on the stalks. It takes about 50 pounds of plants to produce one pound of wax. Harvesting and processing is a labor-intensive venture. Candellila wax is used in many industries, including food and cosmetics. In food, it's used as a coating or in products like chewing gum. In cosmetics, it's used as a stabilizer, to retain moisture or to add firmness and shine to products like, lipstick or lip balm. You will also find it products like mascara and moisturizers.

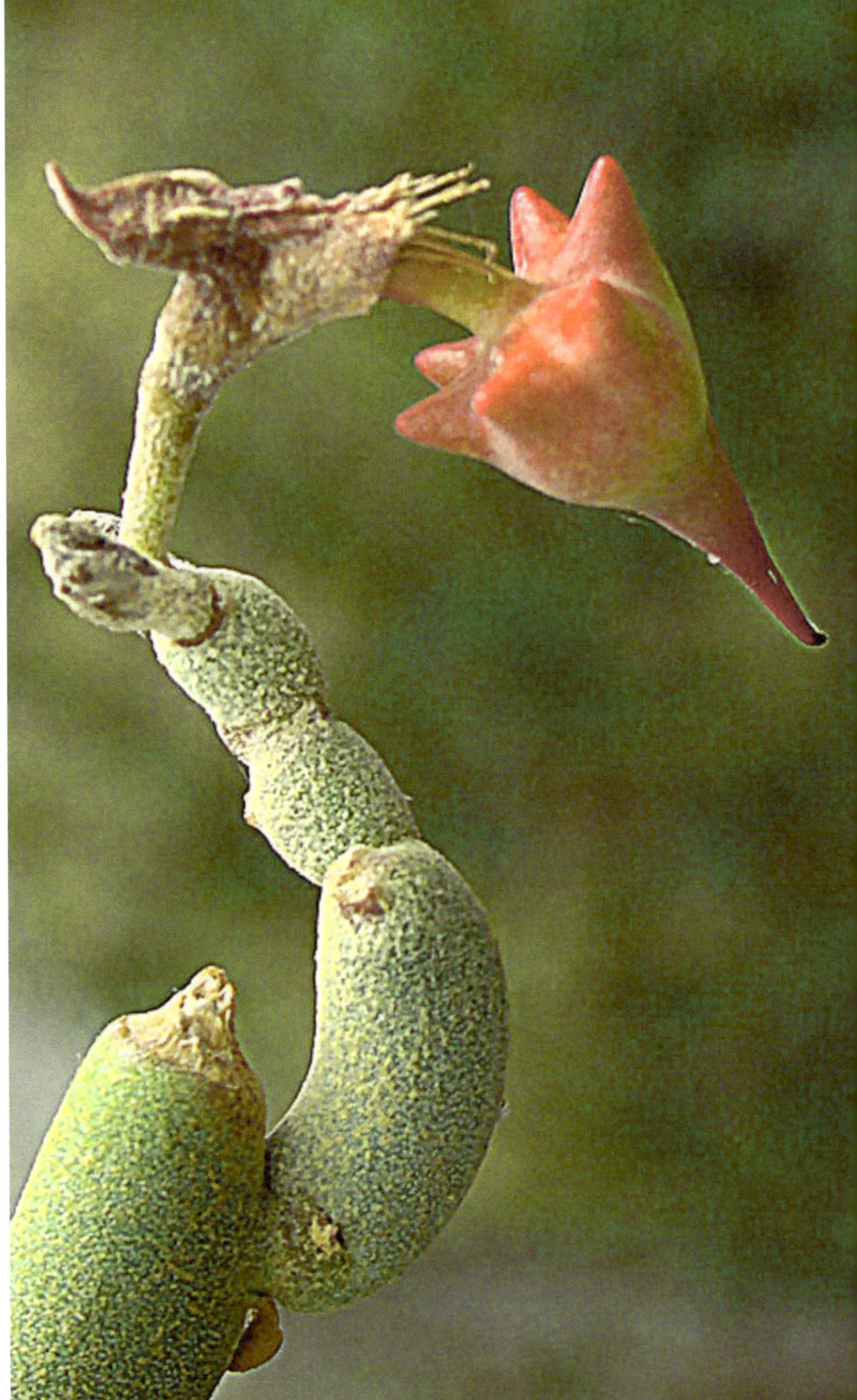

# Castor

The Castor plant produces the seeds from which castor oil is pressed. The castor plant is a subtropical and tropical plant. This oil does an excellent job at maintaining moisture in the skin. Castor oil contains fatty acids and works as a humectant drawing in moisture from the air and retaining moisture on the skin. It's used in soap, lipstick and lip gloss and other cosmetic products.

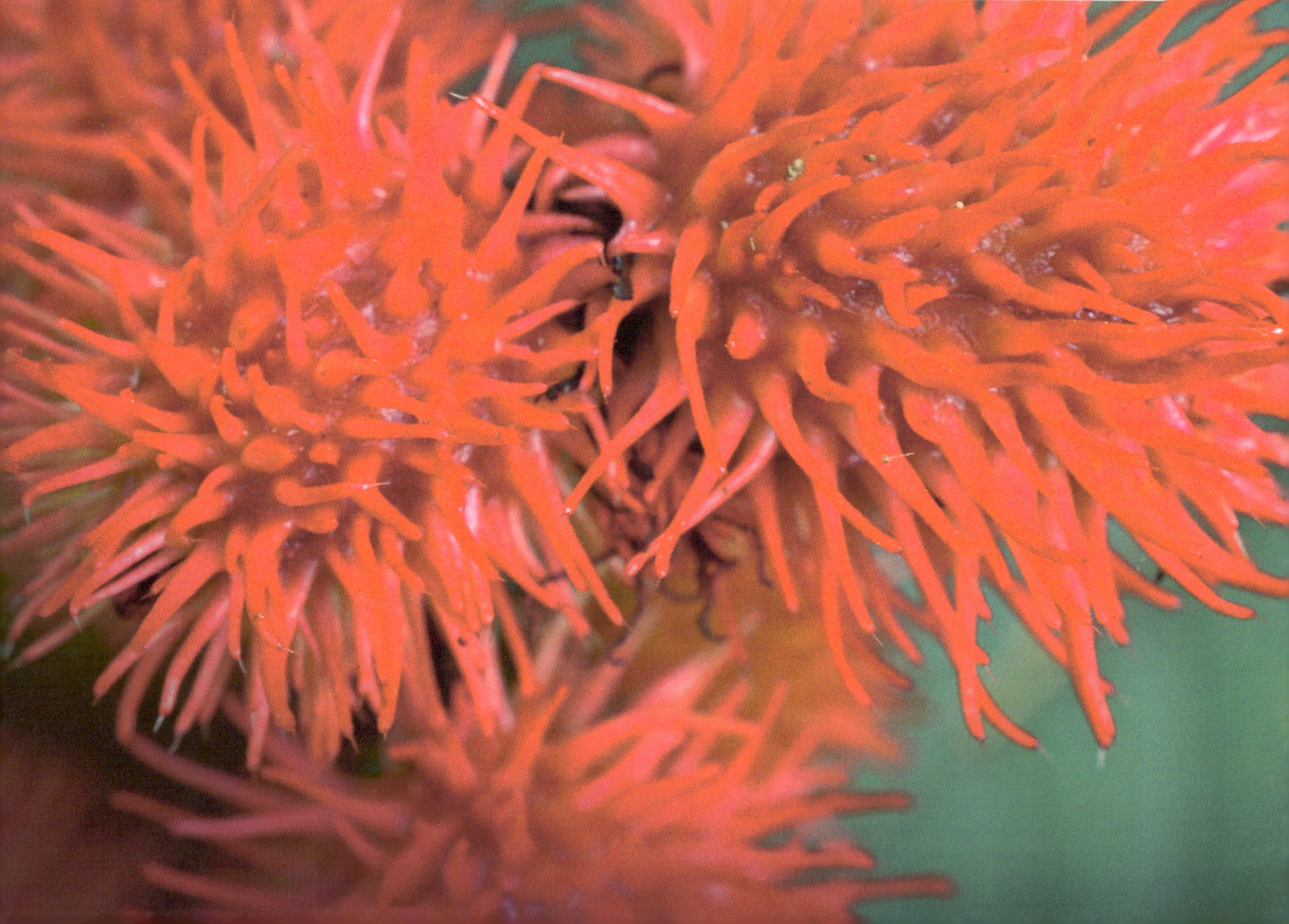

# Diatoms

What's a diatom, you ask? Well, diatoms are microalge, also called phytoplankton, which are single cell organisms. Scientists estimate that there may be up to 2 million different species of diatoms on earth. They are present in bodies of water and even in plants that store water. Their outer cell membrane is primarily comprised of silica. When diatoms die, over time their remains become fossilized. Their fossilized remains are called "Diatomaceous Earth." Diatomite mining is a labor intensive. Once mined, diatomaceous earth is processed for use in a few different industries, one of which is cosmetics. In cosmetics, diatomaceous earth is used in scrub products, moisture and oil control products.

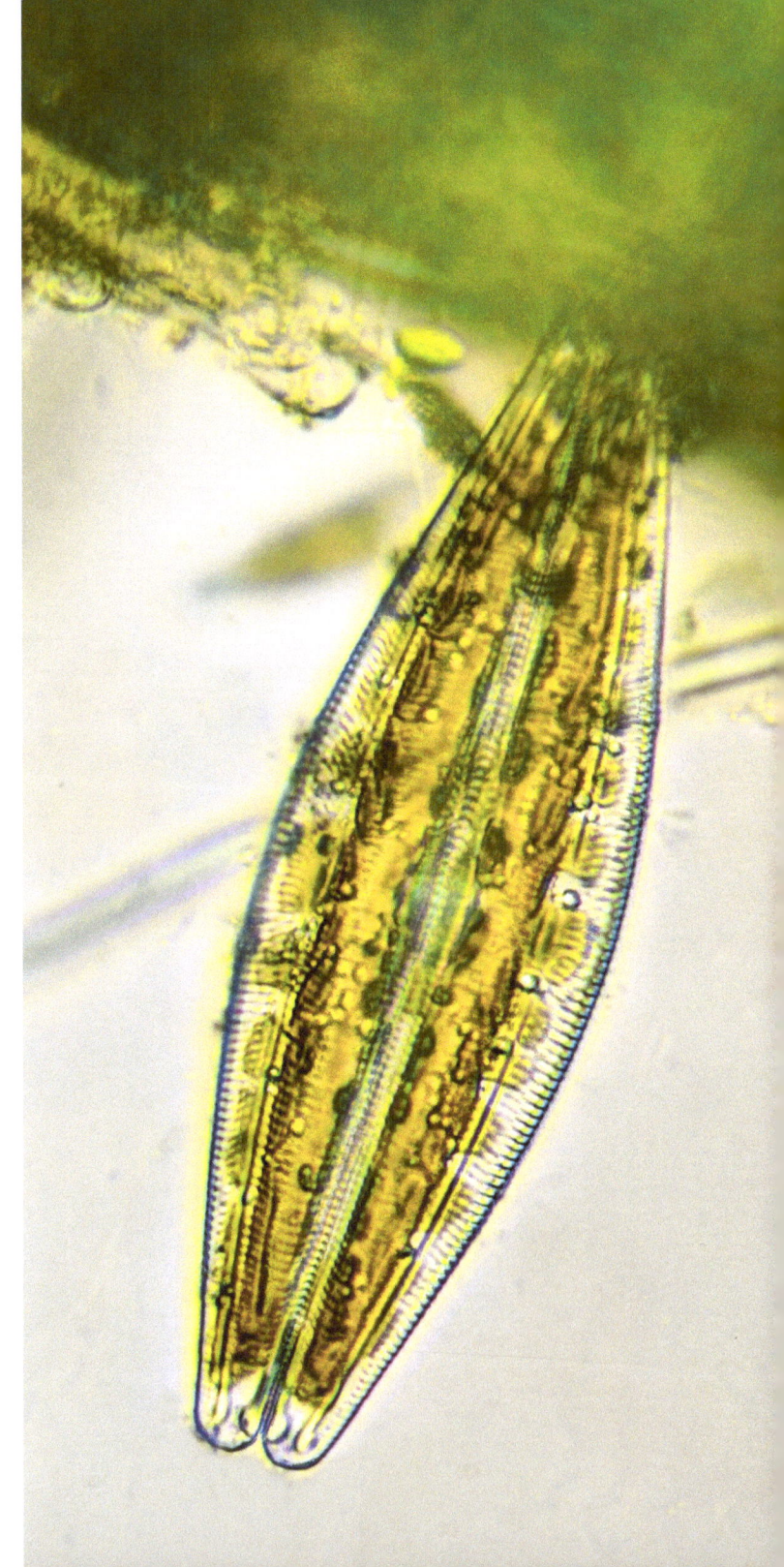

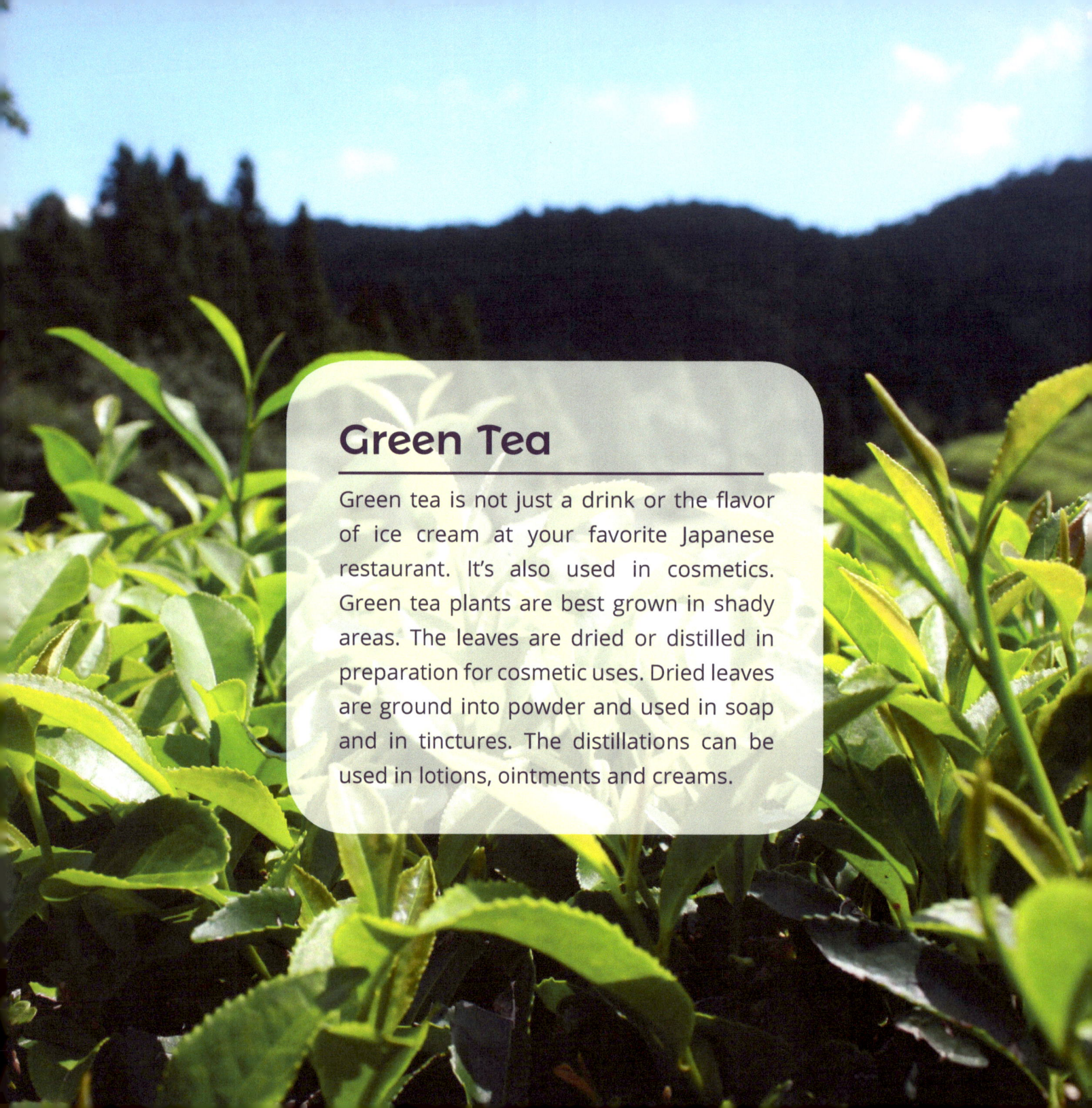

# Green Tea

Green tea is not just a drink or the flavor of ice cream at your favorite Japanese restaurant. It's also used in cosmetics. Green tea plants are best grown in shady areas. The leaves are dried or distilled in preparation for cosmetic uses. Dried leaves are ground into powder and used in soap and in tinctures. The distillations can be used in lotions, ointments and creams.

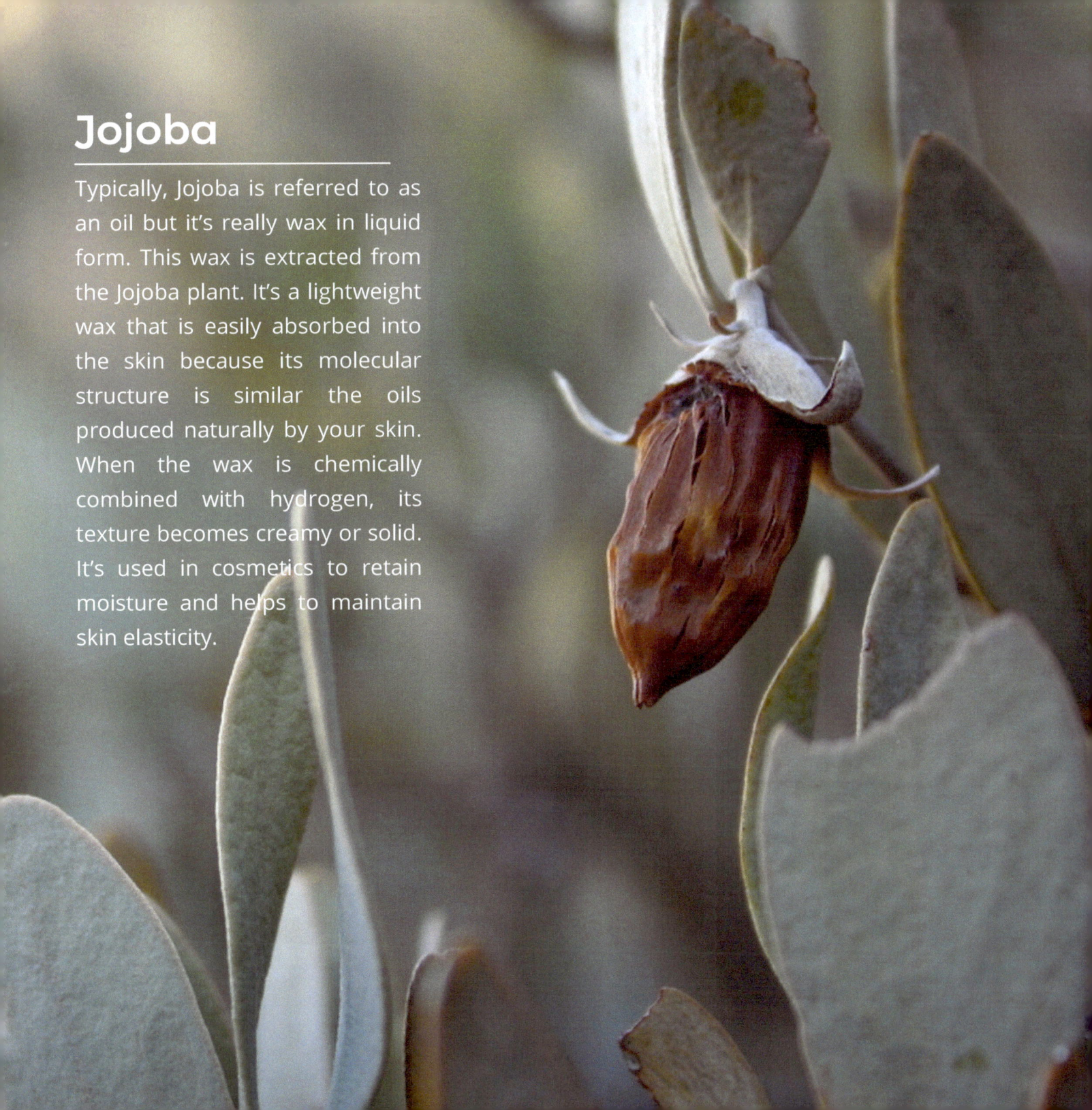

# Jojoba

Typically, Jojoba is referred to as an oil but it's really wax in liquid form. This wax is extracted from the Jojoba plant. It's a lightweight wax that is easily absorbed into the skin because its molecular structure is similar the oils produced naturally by your skin. When the wax is chemically combined with hydrogen, its texture becomes creamy or solid. It's used in cosmetics to retain moisture and helps to maintain skin elasticity.

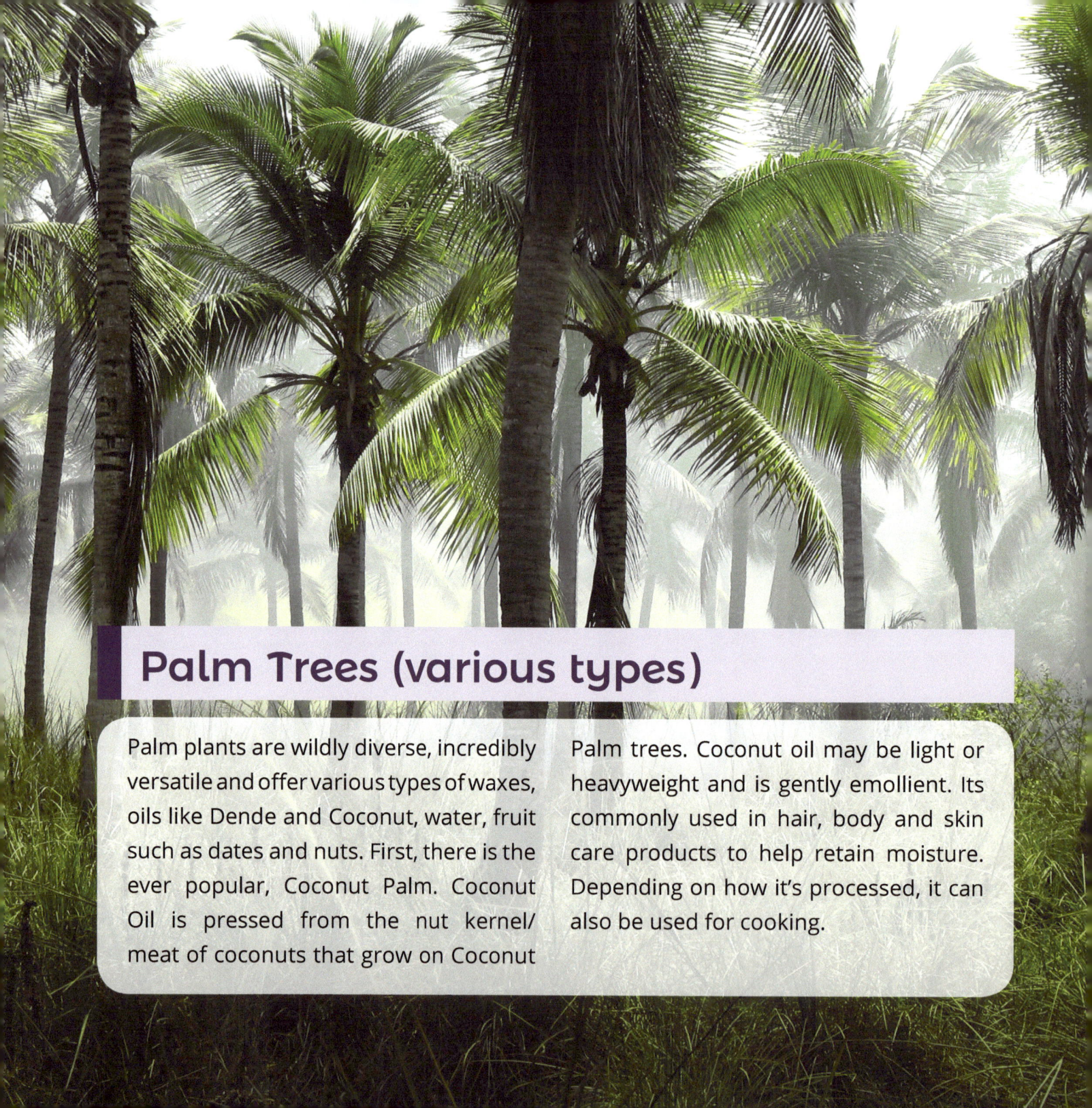

# Palm Trees (various types)

Palm plants are wildly diverse, incredibly versatile and offer various types of waxes, oils like Dende and Coconut, water, fruit such as dates and nuts. First, there is the ever popular, Coconut Palm. Coconut Oil is pressed from the nut kernel/meat of coconuts that grow on Coconut Palm trees. Coconut oil may be light or heavyweight and is gently emollient. Its commonly used in hair, body and skin care products to help retain moisture. Depending on how it's processed, it can also be used for cooking.

## Activated Charcoal

Activated charcoal is also referred to as activated carbon. Activated charcoal is an amazing odor absorber. It's actually a better odor absorber than baking soda. Certain types of activated charcoal have medicinal applications. Activated charcoal is used in toothpaste, deodorant, soap and various other hair, skin and body care products. All that's great, but what does activated charcoal have to do with coconuts, you ask? Most of the activated charcoal powder on the market today is made from coconut husks and shells. The husk is the outer, green-golden husk and the shell is the brown covering between the husk and the nut kernel/meat. The husk and shells are slowly heated to temperatures between 750 degrees and 1300 degrees to produce black activated charcoal. White activated charcoal is most commonly made with wood but it can also be produced using coconut husk and shells. White activated charcoal is made by quickly heating the material to 1800 degrees and quickly cooled with sand to make white activated charcoal.

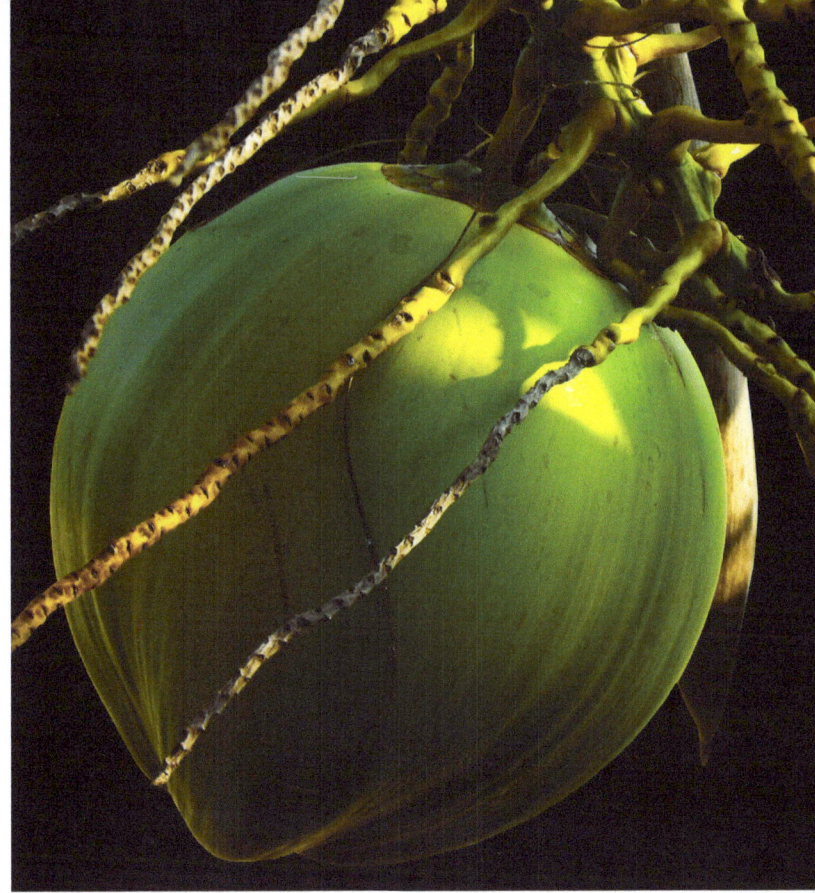

Coconut water is a liquid harvested from inside young or mature coconuts. When it comes to cosmetic use, coconut water is typically dehydrated and the powder residue is used as a cosmetic additive. Coconut water is rich in potassium, however, topical use of potassium is not health benefit, although it is often used in cosmetics.

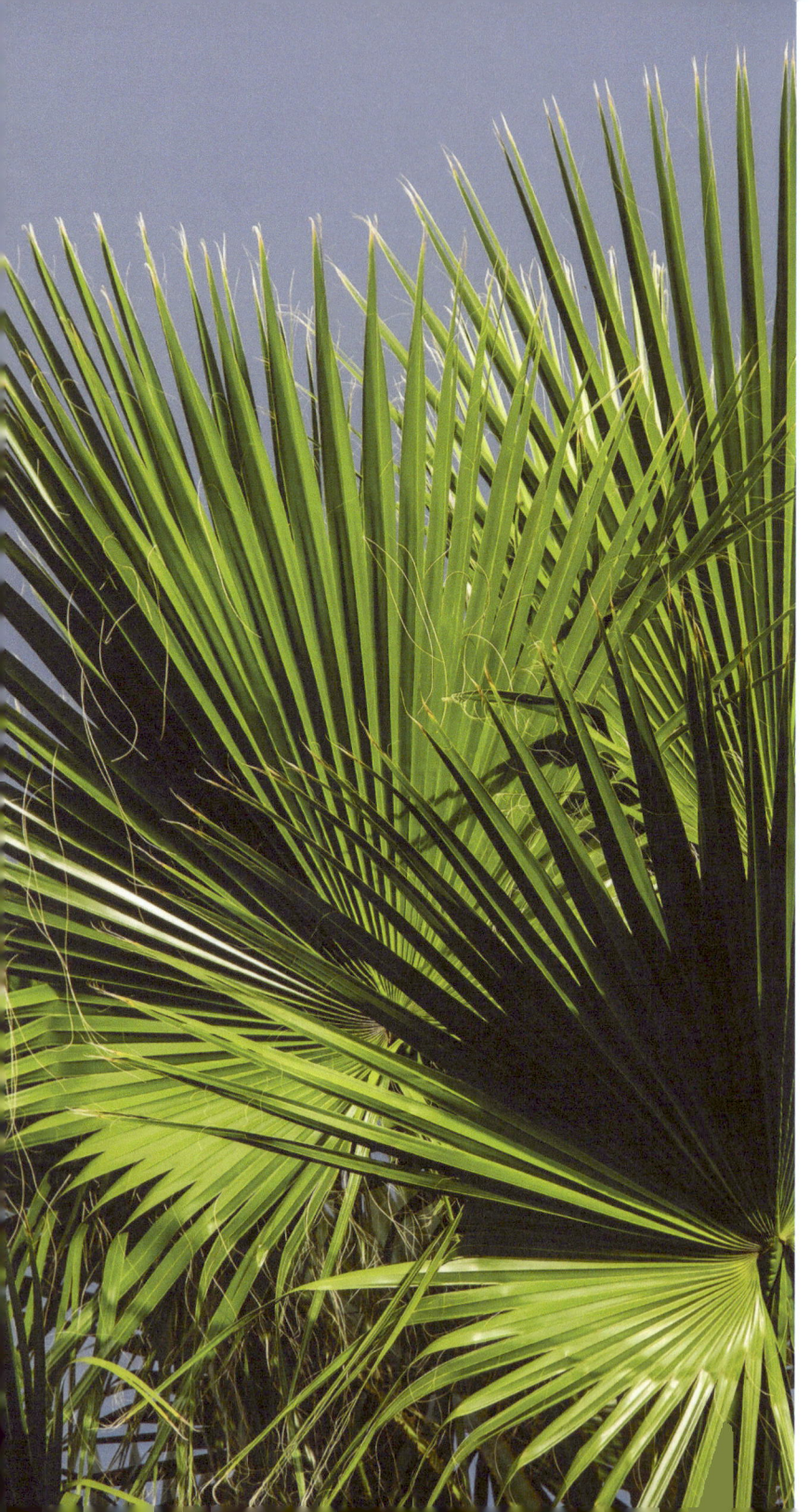

## Carnauba Wax

Carnauba wax is harvested from the leaves of a palm tree which is native to northeastern Brazil. It's also referred to as palm wax and Brazil wax. This wax is hard compared to other plant waxes; yellow in color; and it helps to retain moisture when used in cosmetics. It's processed differently depending on whether it's going to be used for food, cosmetic or industrial applications. In cosmetics, it's used as a stabilizer, thickener or to create a shiny finish in lip products.

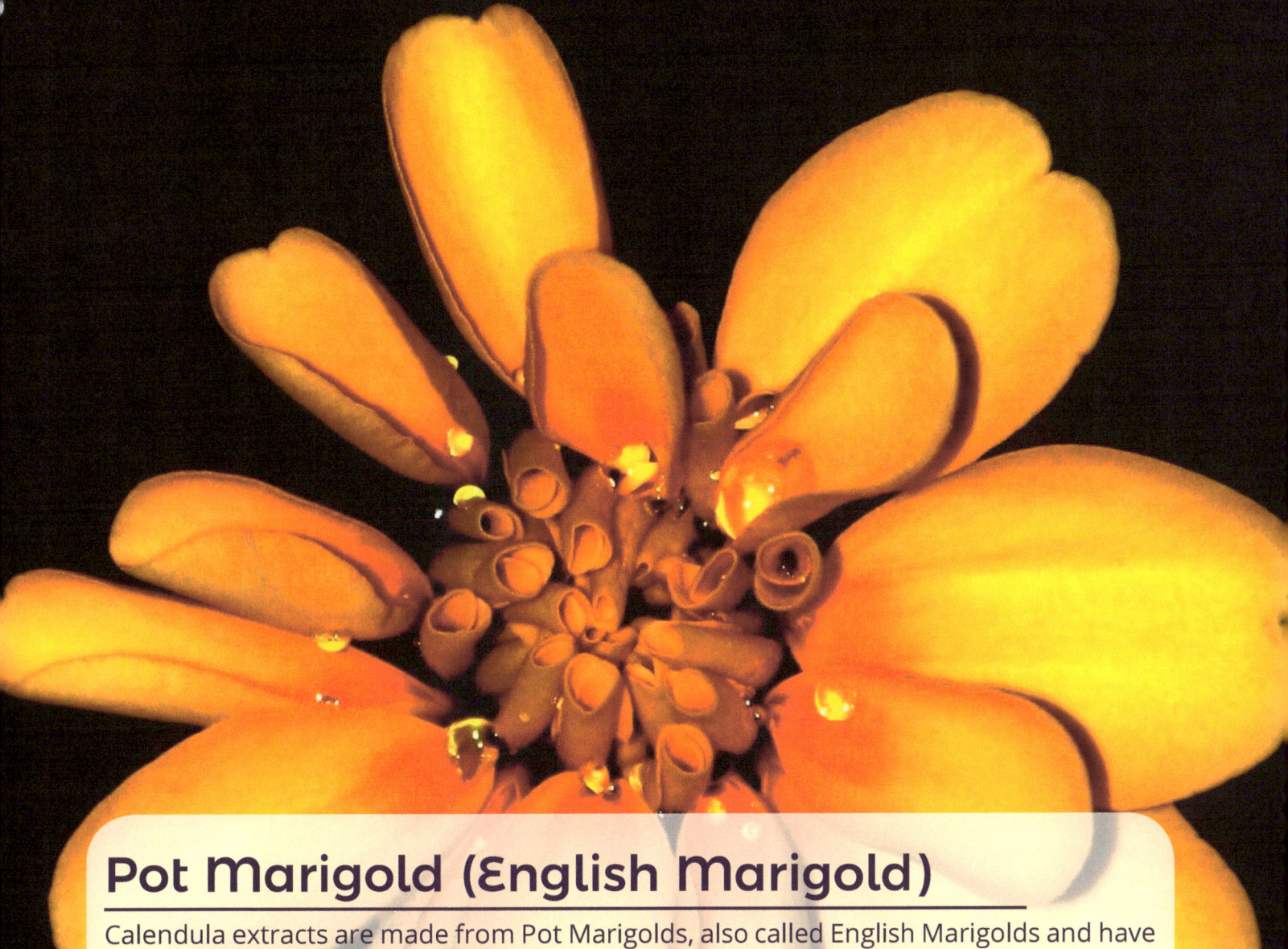

# Pot Marigold (English Marigold)

Calendula extracts are made from Pot Marigolds, also called English Marigolds and have a long history of use in skin care. These are not the most common type of ornamental garden Marigold. The flowers of the Pot Marigold can be vibrant yellow to orange and the petals of the flower are edible. Extracts from the plant are used in infused oils, creams and can also be used as an essential oil. The dried flower petals can also be added to soap, creams and lotions.

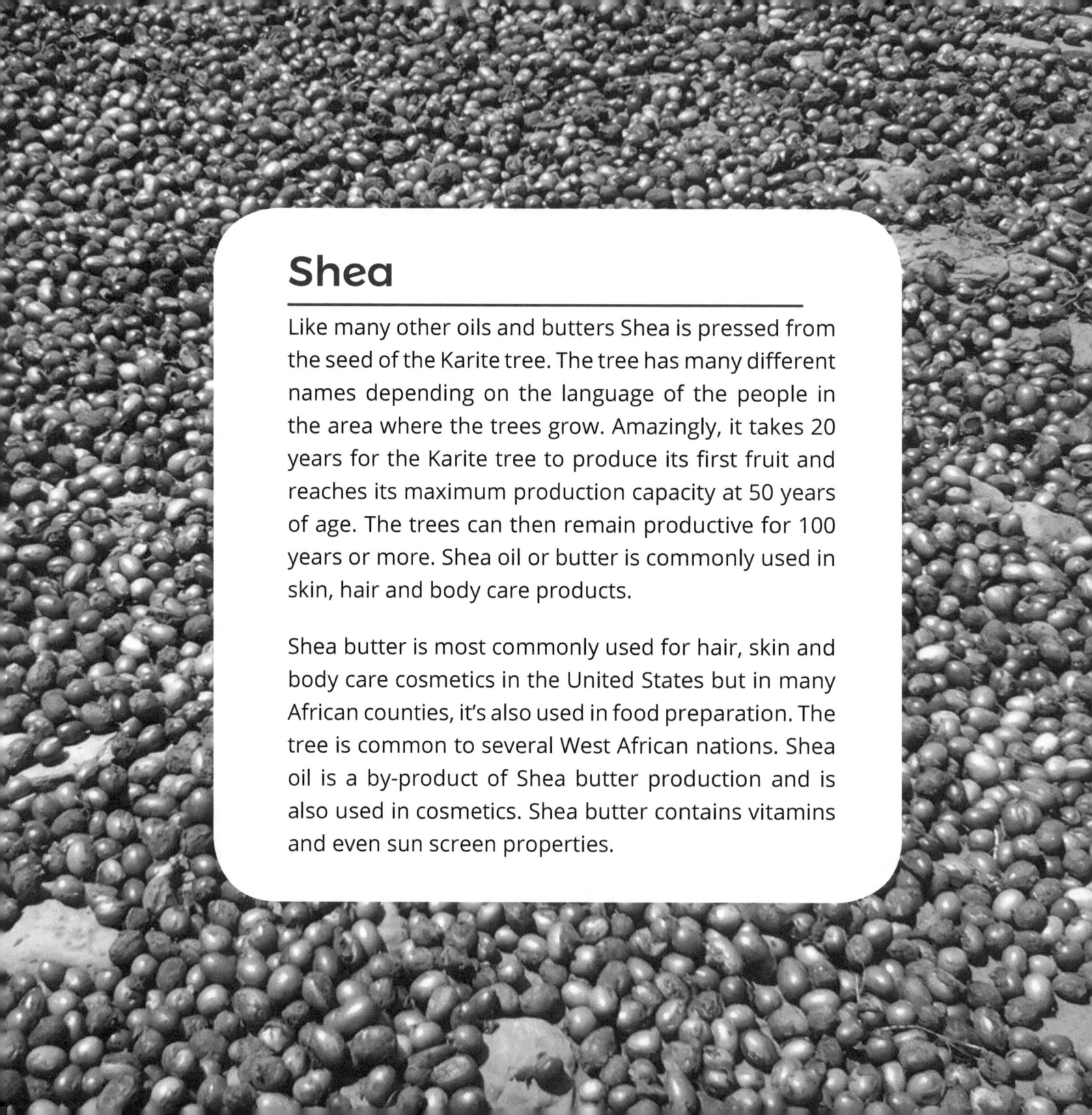

# Shea

Like many other oils and butters Shea is pressed from the seed of the Karite tree. The tree has many different names depending on the language of the people in the area where the trees grow. Amazingly, it takes 20 years for the Karite tree to produce its first fruit and reaches its maximum production capacity at 50 years of age. The trees can then remain productive for 100 years or more. Shea oil or butter is commonly used in skin, hair and body care products.

Shea butter is most commonly used for hair, skin and body care cosmetics in the United States but in many African counties, it's also used in food preparation. The tree is common to several West African nations. Shea oil is a by-product of Shea butter production and is also used in cosmetics. Shea butter contains vitamins and even sun screen properties.

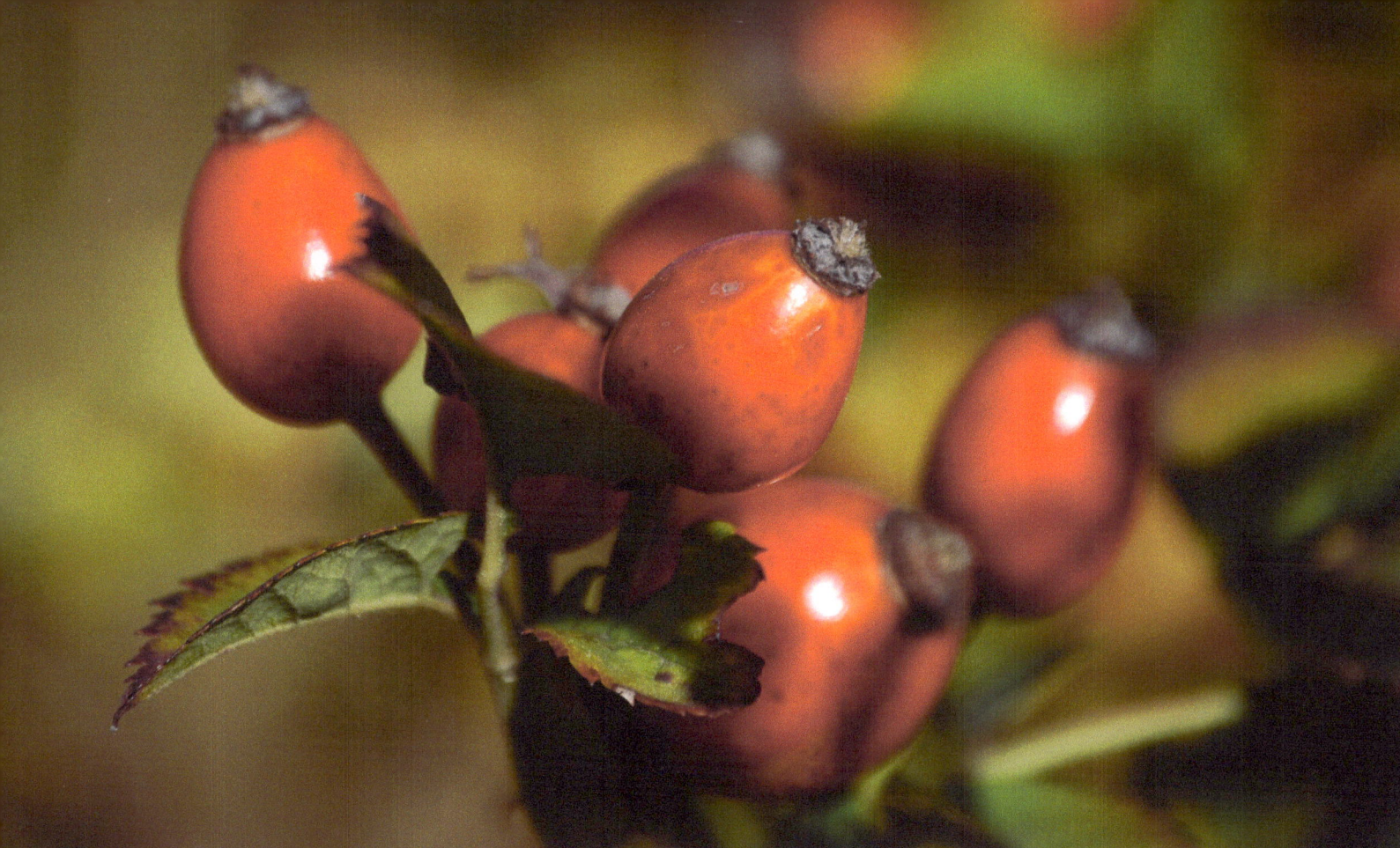

## Rose Hips

The oil pressed from the seeds of wild roses, called Rosa Canina, is extracted for use in skin and hair care products. The rosehip is the fruit of the rose and the seeds are inside the fruit. The fruit can be eaten, used in cosmetics and has a high concentration of vitamin C. The seeds inside the fruit are not edible but the lightweight, dry oil extracted from the seeds is a great skin care ingredient because it contains high levels of fatty acids, omega 3 and 6, all of which promote healthy skin. The shrub can grow up to 14 feet tall. This wild rose grows all over the world now but it's native to western Asia and Europe.

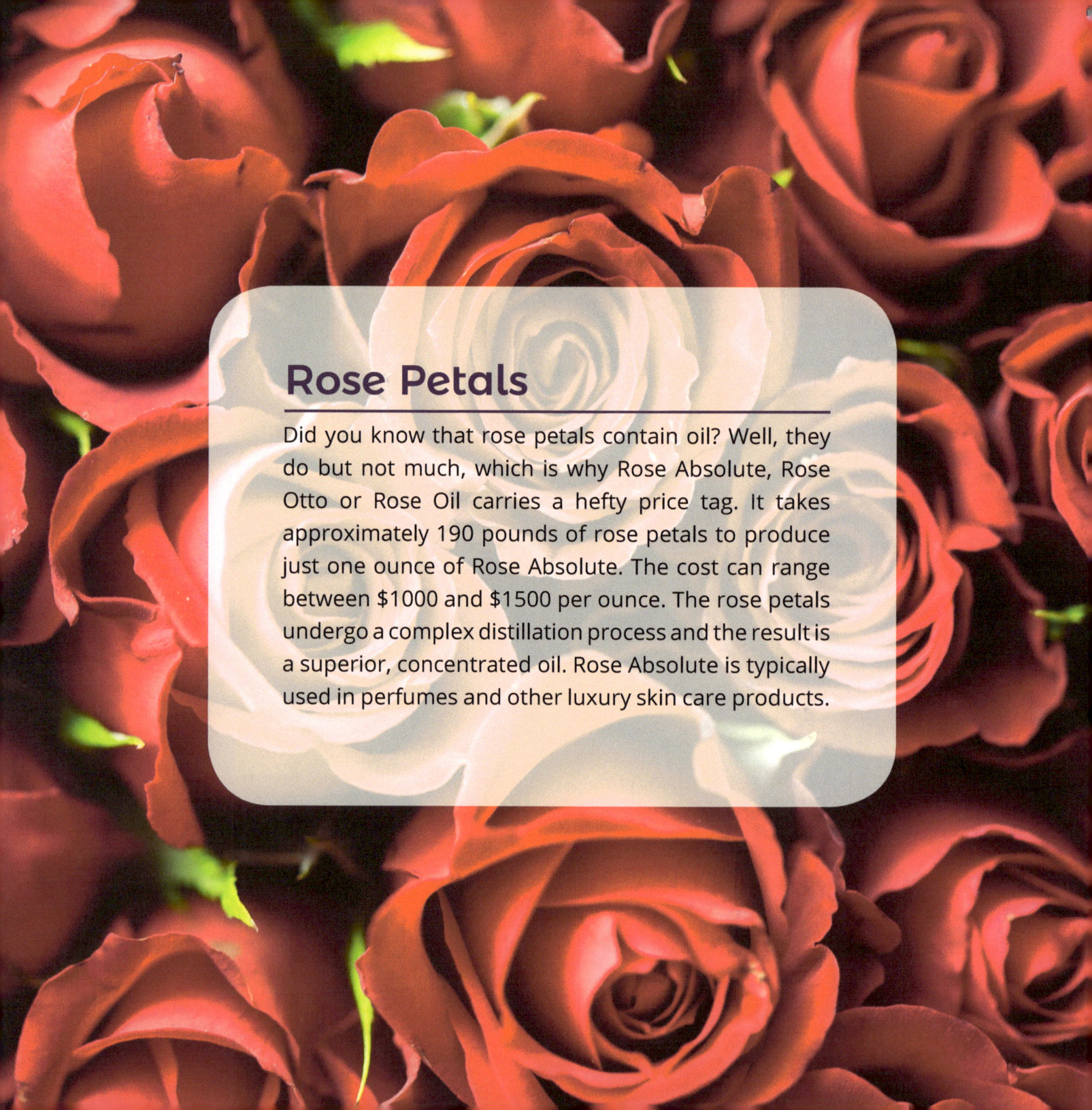

## Rose Petals

Did you know that rose petals contain oil? Well, they do but not much, which is why Rose Absolute, Rose Otto or Rose Oil carries a hefty price tag. It takes approximately 190 pounds of rose petals to produce just one ounce of Rose Absolute. The cost can range between $1000 and $1500 per ounce. The rose petals undergo a complex distillation process and the result is a superior, concentrated oil. Rose Absolute is typically used in perfumes and other luxury skin care products.

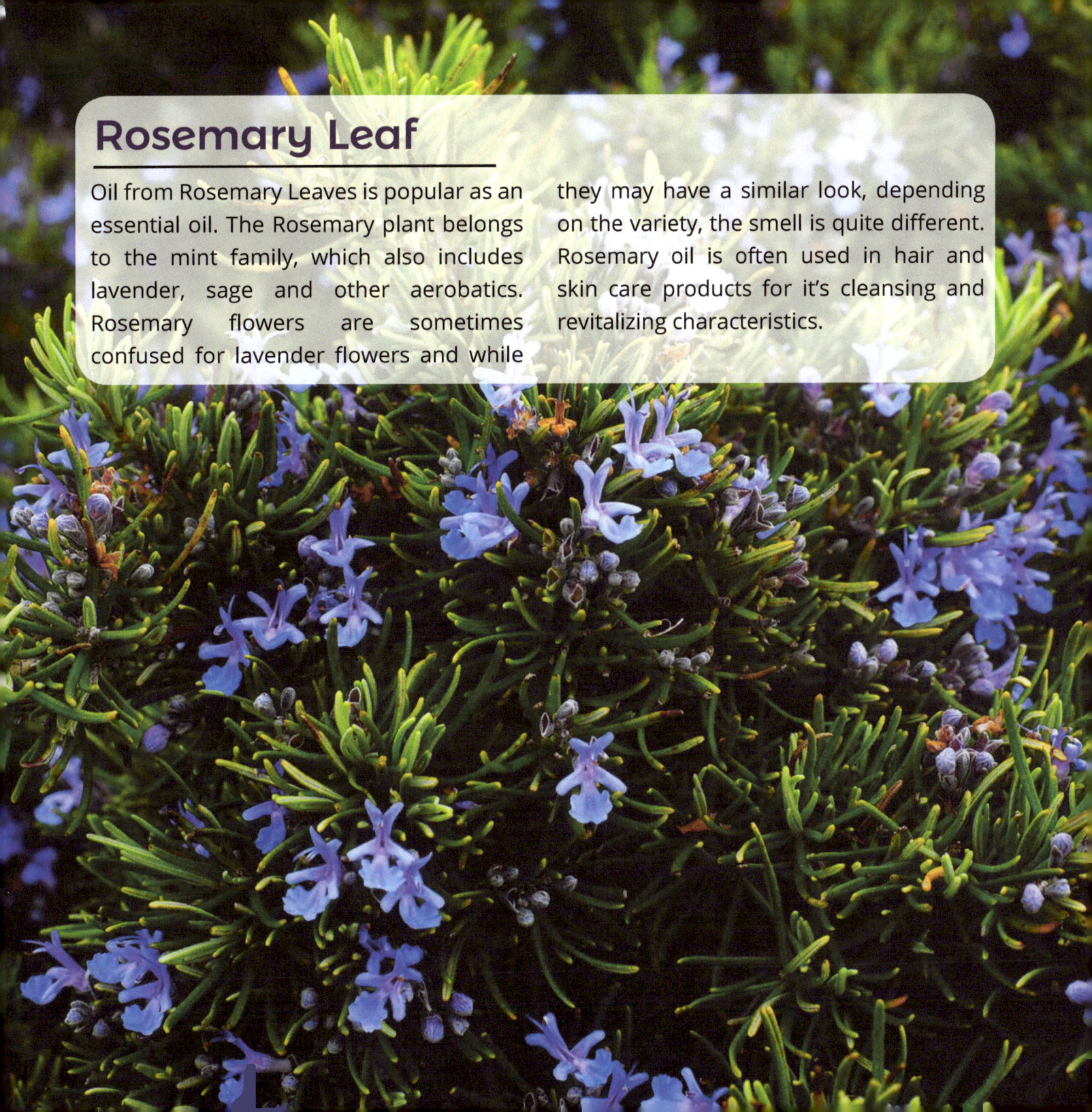

# Rosemary Leaf

Oil from Rosemary Leaves is popular as an essential oil. The Rosemary plant belongs to the mint family, which also includes lavender, sage and other aerobatics. Rosemary flowers are sometimes confused for lavender flowers and while they may have a similar look, depending on the variety, the smell is quite different. Rosemary oil is often used in hair and skin care products for it's cleansing and revitalizing characteristics.

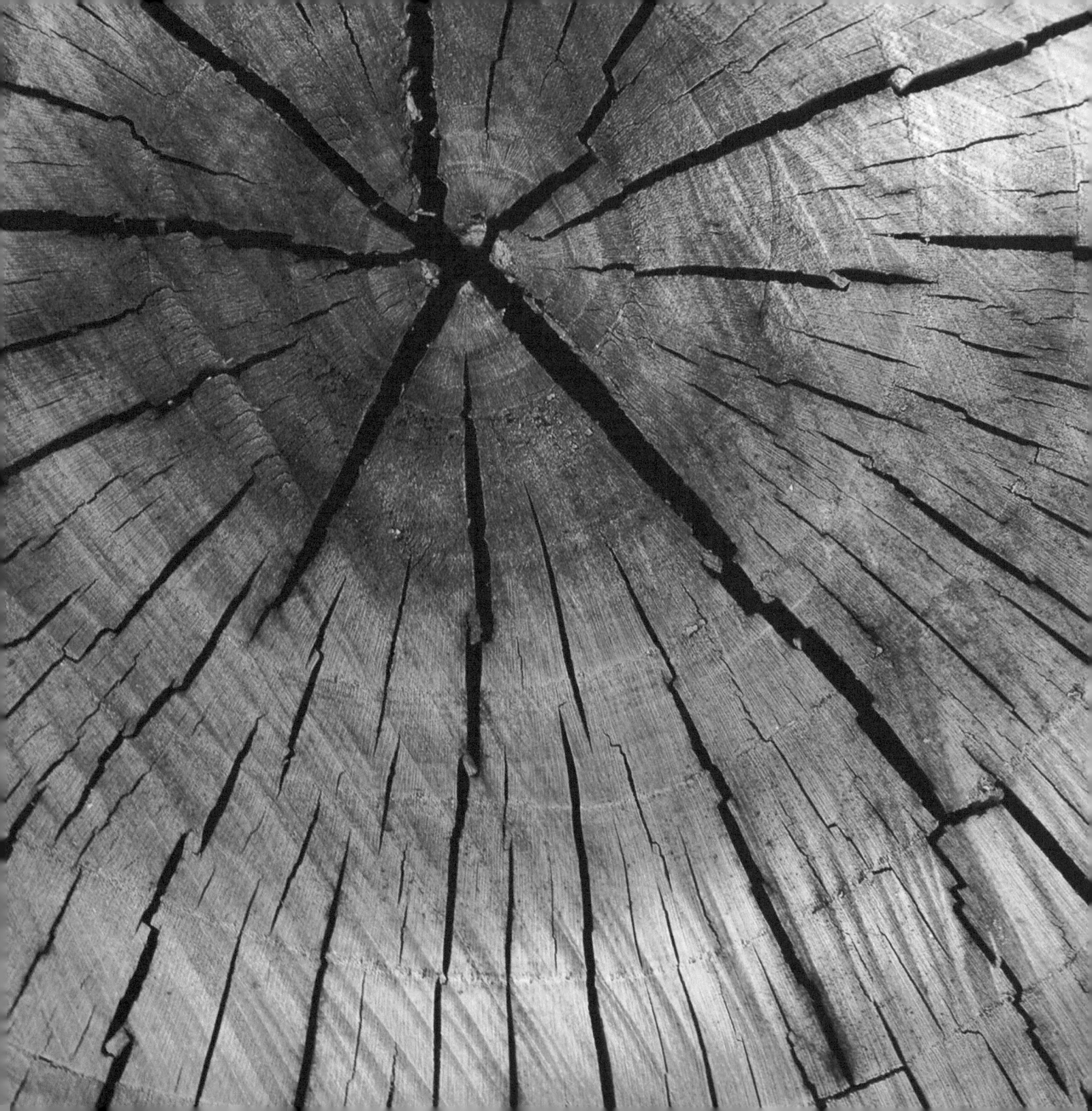

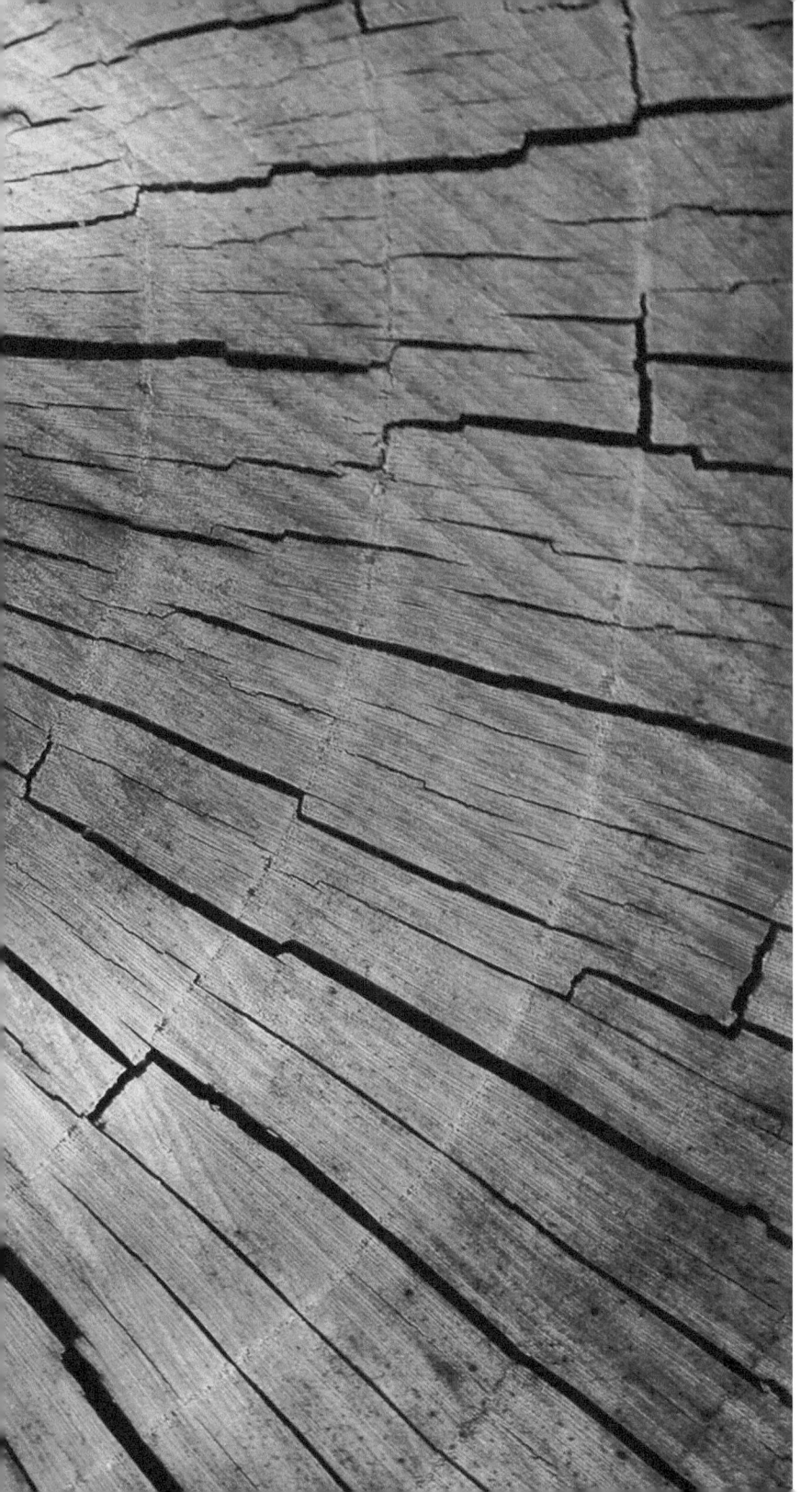

# Wood

Yes, there may be wood in your cosmetics and sometimes your food. It's called Cellulose Gum once it's processed for use in cosmetics or food. Cellulose gum is found in all plants but it's mainly extracted from wood. It's used as a thickener and stabilizer and you'll find it in your shampoo, lotion, hair gel and other types of cosmetic products.

# Sources

Epstein, Samuel S., Gitzgerals, Randall. Healthy Beauty: Your Guide to Ingredients to Avoid and Products You Can Trust. 2010

Jamoke, Hezekia. Cheney, Glen Alan. Dr. Jamoke's Little Book of Hitherto Uncompiled Facts and Curiosities about Bees. CreateSpace Independent Publishing Platform. 2016.

Reed, Valerie, J. Natural Cosmetic Ingredient Dictionary. Unpublished Work

Taylor, Susan C. Brown Skin: Dr. Susan Taylor's Prescription for Flawless Skin, Hair and Nails. Amistad. 2003

Thompson, Kerry., Park, Coco. Korean Beauty Secrets: A Practical Guide to Cutting-Edge Skincare & Makeup. Skyhorse Publishing. 2015

United States Department of Agriculture: Natural Resources Conservation Service. plants.usda.gov

United States Food and Drug Administration. For Consumers

https://www.fda.gov/ForIndustry/ColorAdditives/default.htm (Color Additives)

https://www.fda.gov/ForConsumers/default.htm (For Consumers)

United States Geological Survey: United States Department of the Interior. minerals. usgs.gov

Varinia, M. Michalun. DiNardo, Joseph C. Skin Care and Cosmetic Ingredients Dictionary. Milady. 2014

Winter, Ruth. M.S., A Consumer's Dictionary of Cosmetic Ingredients 6th ed., 2005. Three Rivers Press. New York.

## Image Credit